Patient Care in
Radiography

FOURTH EDITION

Patient Care in

Radiography

Ruth Ann Ehrlich, R.T.R. (ARRT)

Ellen Doble McCloskey, R.N., B.S., M.N.

with 230 illustrations

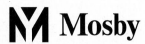 Mosby

St. Louis Baltimore Boston Chicago London Philadelphia Sydney Toronto

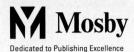
Mosby
Dedicated to Publishing Excellence

Editor: Don E. Ladig
Developmental Editor: Jeanne Rowland
Project Manager: Gayle May Morris
Production Editor: Deborah Vogel
Designer: Jeanne Wolfgeher
Cover Photograph: Custom Medical Stock Photo, Inc.

FOURTH EDITION
Copyright © 1993 by Mosby-Year Book, Inc.

Previous editions copyrighted 1981, 1985, 1989

Printed in the United States of America

Mosby-Year Book, Inc.
11830 Westline Industrial Drive
St. Louis, Missouri 63146

Library of Congress Cataloging-in-Publication Data

Ehrlich, Ruth Ann
     Patient care in radiography / Ruth Ann Ehrlich, Ellen Doble
  McCloskey.—4th ed.
       p.   cm.
     Includes bibliographical references and index.
     ISBN 0-8016-7058-6
     1. Radiography, Medical.   2. Medical personnel and patient.
  I. McCloskey, Ellen Doble.   II. Title.
     [DNLM: 1. Professional-Patient Relations.   2. Radiography.
  3. Technology, Radiologic.   WN 200 E33p]
     RC78.E48   1992
     616.07'572—dc20
     DNLM/DLC   92-49092
     for Library of Congress   CIP

93 94 95 96 97 CL/DC 9 8 7 6 5 4 3 2 1

To
our parents
who supported us with love and encouragement

our children
who helped us by learning patience and self-reliance

our persistence
an often unappreciated virtue

Preface

As the fourth edition of this book becomes a reality, we reaffirm our original purpose: to write a book for radiographers based not on x-ray technique, but on patient care. Our emphasis, as in the three previous editions, is on meeting the physical and emotional needs of patients from a radiographer's point of view.

This is not a technical cookbook. The chapters were not developed in a way that allows them to stand alone. Later chapters build on the vocabulary, concepts, and procedures introduced earlier. Study questions at the ends of the chapters can aid in integrating new information with concepts learned previously. If you are not using the book in chronological order, you will want to use the references to previous chapters so that essential information is not missed.

We expect you to use a good encyclopedic medical dictionary as you read this text. We have defined most new terms as they are introduced, but many of them will be unfamiliar to you and pursuing their definitions will expand your medical knowledge while helping you understand the text itself. The word lists at the beginning of each chapter will also aid in the process of building your medical vocabulary.

While our primary goal is to provide you with a resource on patient care, we are also concerned about you, the caregivers. Please learn and use the self-care concepts underlying the sections on malpractice prevention and body substance precautions, because applying these concepts is as important to you as learning to use a film processor or a pulse oximeter.

Changes in this edition include a detailed discussion of emergency drugs and commonly used medications, a new table and discussion on taking a history, and a completely revised and expanded section on administration of intravenous fluids and medications. As we revised the text, many changes were made in response to the suggestions made by students and instructors. We welcome such suggestions and encourage you to send us your comments.

We are particularly grateful for the information, resources, and photographic opportunities so generously provided by the administration and staff of Oregon Health Sciences University and Southwest Washington Medical Center (SWMC). We especially wish to recognize the photography of Becky Kruse, R.T.R. Becky has illustrated the text from its beginnings in 1978, and continues to provide us with clear pictures and wise counsel.

Our sincere gratitude to Dr. James McAfee, neuroradiologist at SWMC, who not only answered dozens of questions, but provided a thorough and thoughtful review of Chapter 9. Others to whom we are indebted for their help are Joan Daly of the Portland Community College Radiologic Technology faculty, Kathy Pollack, R.T., RDMS, Mary Holt, R.T.R., Jean Overbay, R.T.R., and Philip R. Bennett, J.D.

Our thanks to all of you—students, instructors, and contributors. We could not have done it without you.

Ruth Ann Ehrlich
Ellen Doble McCloskey

Contents

Patient Care in
Radiography

The Radiographer as a Member of the Health Care Team

At the conclusion of this chapter, the student will be able to:

1. State three reasons why a study of professional behavior is important to the radiographer.
2. Describe the radiographer's role in relation to the radiologist, referring physician, hospital administration, nursing personnel, and other hospital staff.
3. List three aspects of self-care that demonstrate responsible behavior by the radiographer.
4. List three ways that a radiographer can contribute to the advancement of radiologic technology.
5. Define *ethics*.
6. Explain the rationale for confidentiality of professional communications.
7. List four patient rights that the radiographer is responsible for protecting.
8. Define the terms *negligence* and *malpractice*.
9. List three specific acts of negligence or malpractice common to radiology departments.
10. Discuss the most frequent circumstances causing patients to initiate litigation.

Vocabulary list

1. assault
2. battery
3. diagnosis
4. ethics
5. false imprisonment
6. intern
7. libel
8. malpractice
9. negligence
10. oncology
11. prognosis
12. radiographer
13. radiography
14. radiologic technologist
15. radiologist
16. resident
17. slander
18. therapy

THE HEALTH CARE TEAM

The most important people in the health care community are the patients. They come to the hospital for help in preserving health or solving health-related problems, and all the efforts of the health care team are directed toward their well-being. As a radiographer, you will be an important member of this team. Therefore, it will be helpful to become acquainted with other team members and their functions in the hospital. Although patients may be seen in physicians' offices, outpatient clinics, and other health care settings, most of your

Table 1-1
Abbreviated table of medical specialties

Specialty	Functions
Anesthesiologist	Administers anesthetics and monitors the patient during surgery
Dermatologist	Diagnoses and treats conditions and diseases of the skin
Emergency department physician	Specializes in trauma and emergency situations; a triage expert in disaster situations
Family practice physician	Treats individuals and families in the context of daily life
Gastroenterologist	Diagnoses and treats diseases of the gastrointestinal tract
Geriatrician	Specializes in problems and diseases of elderly persons
Gynecologist	Treats problems and diseases of the female reproductive system
Internist	Specializes in diseases of the internal organs
Neurologist	Specializes in functions and disorders of the nervous system
Obstetrician	Specializes in pregnancy, labor, delivery, and immediate postpartum care
Oncologist	Specializes in tumor identification and treatment
Ophthalmologist	Diagnoses and treats problems and diseases of the eye
Otorhinolaryngologist	Specializes in conditions of the ear, nose, and throat
Pathologist	Specializes in the scientific study of the alterations in the body caused by disease and death
Pediatrician	Treats and diagnoses children
Psychiatrist	Specializes in diagnosis, treatment, and prevention of mental illness
Radiologist	Specializes in diagnosis by means of medical imaging
Surgeons	
Abdominal	Specializes in surgery of the abdominal cavity
Neurological	Specializes in surgery of the brain, spinal cord, and peripheral nervous system
Orthopedic	Diagnoses and treats problems of the musculoskeletal system
Plastic	Restores or improves the appearance and function of exposed body parts
Thoracic	Specializes in problems of the chest
Urologic	Diagnoses and treats problems of the urinary tract and the male reproductive system

clinical experience will occur in a hospital, which is the setting on which this book is focused.

Physicians

The patient may come directly to the emergency room or may be sent to the hospital by a doctor, the *referring physician.* On admission, the referring physician may serve as the *attending physician,* continuing to provide direction for care, or another physician may be assigned. In either case, the attending physician is responsible for assessing each patient's needs and prescribing therapeutic procedures designed to promote health.

The attending physician may determine that the expertise of one or more specialists would be helpful in the patient's diagnosis or treatment. The patient might then be referred to the specialist for consultation. A list of specialty areas is found in Table 1-1. This list will assist you in learning the hospital language.

Hospital staff

The physicians who practice in the hospital form the *medical staff.* This group may also include interns and residents, depending on the institution's size and organization. The hospital is governed by an executive board, which establishes policies, goals, and financial plans and hires the director or administrator. One of the Board's responsibilities is to extend the privilege of staff membership to qualified physician applicants and to organize the staff to cooperate in making the rules that govern their activities. Many of these rules relate to standards of care and medical records.

In addition, the administration must see that suitable facilities and equipment are provided and that a staff of well-trained professional, technical, and support personnel is present. Fig. 1-1 shows a typical organizational structure common for hospitals and the lines of authority and responsibility that form a *chain of command* for the health care team.

The director may be assisted by one or more assistant administrators with clearly defined areas of responsibility for several departments. They do not need specific training and experience in the areas under their direction because their expertise is in health care management. They rely on department super-

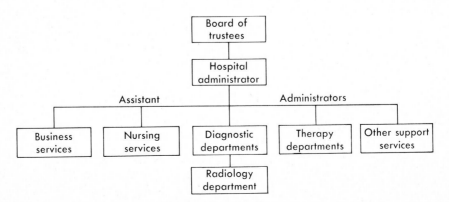

Fig. 1-1. Simplified example of hospital organizational chart.

visors for decisions and communications at the level where specialization is required.

Each department has a chief or supervisor whose education and expertise relate directly to the area of responsibility. For example, the supervisor of the hospital pharmacy is a registered pharmacist, whereas the supervisor of the radiology department is usually a radiographer. Each supervisor leads a group of skilled employees who carry out the department's goals.

Some departments meet patient needs directly. Nursing service is a good example. It provides patient care by implementing nursing care decisions, carries out physician orders within the framework of hospital policies, and communicates plans for patient care and physician orders to other departments. Some typical hospital departments are listed in Table 1-2. It is helpful to categorize some of them according to whether their functions are diagnostic, meaning related to identification of patient problems, or therapeutic, meaning devoted to treatment. Still other departments serve patients indirectly by providing support services, such as purchasing, central supply, and laundry. Social service departments may support patients and their families by providing a hospital chaplain or trained counselor. These departments also coordinate with other agencies and services as needed when a patient is discharged or transferred. Many hospitals also have auxiliary groups consisting of volunteers who minister to special needs of patients and their families. Very large institutions often include departments of research and education as well as separate departments or clinics for providing outpatient services. The names of many departments and the way they fit into the chain of command vary with the institution's size and its management philosophy. It is useful to study the organizational chart of the hospital where you are employed.

Few patients use the services of all departments, but the well-being of most patients requires the cooperative efforts of many team members. One may gain a better understanding of how the team functions by focusing attention on one patient.

Table 1-2

Some typical hospital departments

Direct patient services			
General	**Diagnostic**	**Therapeutic**	**Support services**
Admitting	Electrocardiography	Dietary	Bookkeeping
Emergency	(ECG)	Respiratory therapy	Housekeeping
Nursing service	Electroencephalography	Occupational therapy	Laundry
Social services	(EEG)	Physical therapy	Library
	Nuclear medicine	Radiation oncology	Maintenance
	Pathology (medical laboratories)	Surgery	Medical records
			Personnel
	Radiology		Purchasing
	Ultrasonography		

Mrs. Cohen was admitted to the hospital with severe back pain following a motor vehicle accident. Her family physician, Dr. Evans, requested an x-ray examination of the spine to aid in diagnosis and the planning of an effective course of treatment. The examination request was actually a referral to a specialist, the radiologist, for diagnostic consultation. Dr. Evans wrote the order in Mrs. Cohen's chart, and a nurse made arrangements for the procedure.

Mrs. Cohen and her chart were brought to the radiology department by a transportation orderly. The radiographer greeted her, explained the procedure, and performed the examination, using the chart to confirm the order and note any special or helpful information. Clean linen used for the examination was provided by the hospital laundry. Several members of the radiology department staff assisted by processing the paper work, developing the film, and helping to move the patient. A supervising radiographer checked the films to see that they met the standards of the radiologist, the department, and the hospital. Mrs. Cohen was then returned by the orderly to the care of the nursing service.

The radiologist studied the radiographs and dictated a report of the findings. A medical transcriber typed the report, and a clerk filed the films. A copy of the report was placed in the chart, and a second copy was sent to Dr. Evans, who was then able to confirm the diagnosis.

Therapy was implemented with the help of other team members. For Mrs. Cohen, this included a prescription from the hospital pharmacy and several trips to the physical therapy department.

Members of the business office staff used information from the various departments to prepare the billing. Copies were sent to Mrs. Cohen and to her insurance company. The payment received helped support the many services rendered by the hospital, including the purchase of x-ray film and the radiographer's salary.

Mrs. Cohen's chart was reviewed by a medical staff committee in a random sampling to see that hospital regulations had been followed and to gather statistics about hospital services. The chart was then filed for future reference, since it may be needed again to assist in her care. The radiographs, which are part of the medical record, were also kept on file.

Mrs. Cohen's case is a simplified representation of a hospital stay. How many departments shared responsibility for her care? What types of communication were required to coordinate the team's efforts? Were any of the team members unnecessary or unimportant?

Radiology services

Radiology provides various diagnostic services that relate directly to the patient. The administrative structure is diagrammed in Fig. 1-2. Radiologists, who are members of the medical staff, serve as consultants in one or more of the imaging modalities in radiology. The line of responsibility for radiologists is through the medical staff organization. Radiologists play a major role in establishing standards of care and technical quality within the department, in addition to performing many examinations with the assistance of radiographers (Fig. 1-3). Each examination must be interpreted by a radiologist and the information provided to the referring physician.

The radiology services in a modern hospital are divided among several departments under the supervision of a *radiology manager*. This person works with the radiologists to establish policies and budgets for the various imaging depart-

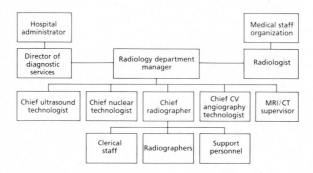

Fig. 1-2. Typical organizational structure of the radiology department.

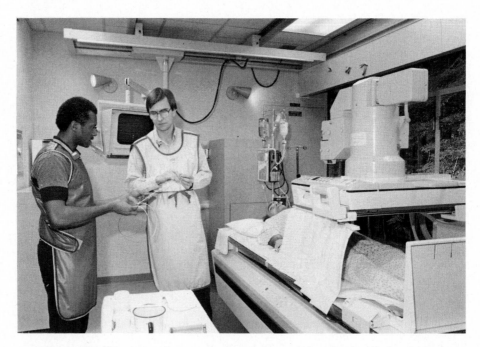

Fig. 1-3. Radiologists perform many examinations with radiographers' assistance.

ments and supervises the chief technologists in each area, including radiography, nuclear medicine, ultrasound, cardiovascular angiography, computed tomography (CT), and magnetic resonance imaging (MRI). This text primarily focuses on the radiography department. Chapter 9 provides an introduction to the other modalities and corresponding aspects of patient care.

The *chief radiographer,* or chief x-ray technologist, supervises the day-to-day activities in the radiography department. He or she also schedules the staff of radiographers and support personnel in this area and orders the necessary supplies. Division of responsibility between the chief technologist and the radiology manager varies with the institution. The chief technologist is often promoted from the ranks of staff radiographers because of both technical expertise and supervisory capability.

Staff radiographers report directly to the chief technologist. In practice, they also work and communicate directly with radiologists rather than along the established chain of command.

Good communication systems depend on the ability of all team members to relay information systematically, which prevents essential details from being overlooked. As you begin to understand team members' responsibilities, you will appreciate the cooperation and communication lines that help the team to function smoothly.

PROFESSIONAL RESPONSIBILITIES
Credentialing and continuing education

Credentials are documents that verify qualifications and aid in quality assurance in a professional setting. Credentials of importance to radiographers include accreditation, registration, licensure, certification, and permits.

Institutional credentials. *Accreditation* is a process that applies to institutions and results in documents that attest to the attainment of certain minimum standards. Hospitals seek accreditation by the Joint Commission for the Accreditation of Healthcare Organizations (JCAHO), which indicates that the institution meets criteria for equipment, staff, safety, funding, management, and patient care. This credential is required for the hospital to receive Medicare payments and for insurance payments by many private carriers.

Accreditation of colleges and universities is the province of state and regional agencies. This credential attests to certain standards of education in accredited institutions. It is the basis for acknowledging the value of the diplomas granted as well as the value of credits transferred from one institution to another.

Two national agencies are particularly important to radiographers because they set standards and are involved in the credentialing of radiologic technology programs. The Joint Review Committee on Education in Radiologic Technology (JRCERT) is made up of members appointed by the American College of Radiology (ACR), the Association of Educators in Radiological Sciences (AERS), and the American Society of Radiologic Technologists (ASRT). JRCERT provides specific guidelines for accreditation of radiologic technology programs, conducts inspections, and makes effective recommendations regarding accreditation. For 15 years the accrediting agency has been the Committee on Allied Health Education and Accreditation (CAHEA), a division of the American Medical Association (AMA). The AMA has announced plans to dissolve CAHEA. A task force has been appointed to create a new agency that will provide accreditation to allied health programs in the future.

The accreditation process for any institution, whether hospital or school, involves periodic "self-study" in which the institution assesses its goals, strengths, and weaknesses and documents how it meets the established criteria for quality in its field. This activity is followed by an on-site visit by representatives of the accrediting agency, during which interviews, physical surveys, and review of documents are used to assess the institution. Accreditation provides incentive for the institution to strive for excellence while assuring the consumer of the quality of services offered.

Individual credentials.   In the field of radiologic technology, such credentials as registration, permits, certificates, and licenses refer to documents that attest to the qualifications of *individuals*.

The American Registry of Radiologic Technologists (ARRT) is a national organization that, as with the JRCERT, is composed of appointees from both the ACR and the ASRT. The ARRT establishes minimum standards for application for registration; that is, the applicant must be a high-school graduate or equivalent and must have completed an approved program in radiologic technology. The ARRT provides a qualifying examination and entitles the applicants who pass to use the designation *radiologic technologist* (RT) in association with their names. The ARRT conducts specialty examinations in radiography (R), nuclear medicine (NM), radiation therapy (T), and diagnostic medical sonography (RDMS) and permits use of these abbreviations with the RT designation. Registration by ARRT is recognized nationally and to some degree internationally as a standard qualification to practice radiologic technology. It is a prerequisite for employment in this field by most accredited institutions. Registration must be renewed biannually by means of paying a nominal fee and completing a questionnaire documenting current employment status and eligibility for renewal. In the near future, eligibility for renewal probably will also be based on proof of continuing education. Registration by the ARRT is an important goal for student radiographers.

Licensure refers to the granting of "official permission" and is a prerogative of state governments. All states have laws requiring driver's licenses and licenses to practice medicine and nursing. Some states also have license requirements to practice radiologic technology. State licensure of radiologic technology began in the 1970s with new laws in New York, New Jersey, and California. Many other states followed this lead. The most recent at this writing is the state of Washington in 1992. Licensure laws vary greatly among the individual states. Many states grant a license to any person registered by ARRT who applies and pays a fee. Other states (e.g., Hawaii) require that a state examination be passed. The new Washington state law requires ARRT registration and proof that an approved 7-hour course on human immunodeficiency virus (HIV) infection has been completed. Other states (e.g., Oregon) require proof of continuing education for license renewal.

Many states grant licenses by means of reciprocity; that is, a license in one state is granted on the basis of prior qualification to practice in another state. Some states enter into reciprocity agreements to facilitate movement of professionals between states where similar qualifications prevail. Radiographers must be aware of the requirements of the states in which they wish to practice and prepare in advance to meet the necessary criteria. Examinations may be offered infrequently, and this could result in a delay in obtaining a license to practice.

Some states issue *permits* to practice radiologic technology under limited circumstances or in limited scope. These permits do not require the same high standards necessary for registration or licensure. Limited permits may allow a public health nurse to take chest radiographs or an orthopedic assistant to take extremity radiographs while helping with application of a cast. Usually an applicant must demonstrate knowledge of radiation safety and technical expertise in a limited area of radiography to obtain a permit.

Certification, as contrasted with licensure or registration, usually means that an individual has completed a limited course of study in a specific area. A certificate may be required of the radiographer to obtain a license (e.g., the HIV Infection Instruction Certificate required by the state of Washington) or *in addition to* registration and/or licensure. Typical examples are the periodic cardiopulmonary resuscitation (CPR) certification, which is required of all patient care personnel in most hospital settings, and venipuncture certification, which may be either a state or institutional requirement for all personnel drawing blood or administering intravenous fluids and medications. Certification requirements provide incentive to maintain competencies and document qualifications.

Knowing the credentials required in a given situation and maintaining current credentials are important professional responsibilities. Violation of state licensure laws may result in fines and imprisonment.

In radiologic technology, as in any rapidly changing technological field, continuing education is essential to stay abreast of current trends and maintain competencies. This also is an important professional responsibility.

Some states now require regular formalized continuing education as a qualification to practice radiologic technology. If you are required to provide evidence of continuing education because of certification or licensing requirements, be sure to determine in advance whether the education you plan to receive is approved and accredited for this purpose. Also, be sure to keep an accurate record of your continuing education activities and any documentation of participation that you receive. Documentation is valuable even if it is not immediately required. It may help in qualifying for a promotion or a new position or assist your professional advancement in unforeseeable ways.

Failure to maintain competency, licensure, registration, or required certification places the employer and the employee at risk and may result in loss of employment and professional reputation.

The code of ethics

Ethics are defined as moral principles or values. With respect to a profession, ethics imply rules or standards that govern the conduct of its members. The Code of Ethics of the American Society of Radiologic Technologists is on pp. 10 and 11.

Code of Ethics for the Profession of Radiologic Technology

Principle 1. The Radiologic Technologist functions efficiently and effectively, demonstrating conduct and attitudes reflecting the profession.

    1.1   Responds to patient needs.

    1.2   Performs tasks competently.

    1.3   Supports colleagues and associates in providing quality patient care.

Principle 2. The Radiologic Technologist acts to advance the principal objective of the profession to provide services to humanity with full respect for the dignity of humankind.

    2.1   Participates in and actively supports the professional organizations for radiologic technology.

    2.2   Acts as a representative for the profession and the tenets for which it stands.

    2.3   Serves as an advocate of professional policy and procedure to colleagues and associates in the health care delivery system.

Principle 3. The Radiologic Technologist provides service to patients without discrimination.

    3.1   Exhibits no prejudice for sex, race, creed, religion.

    3.2   Provides service without regard to social or economic status.

    3.3   Delivers care unrestricted by concerns for personal attributes, nature of the disease or illness.

Principle 4. The Radiologic Technologist practices technology founded on scientific basis.

    4.1   Applies theoretical knowledge and concepts in the performance of tasks appropriate to the practice.

    4.2   Utilizes equipment and accessories consistent with the purpose for which it has been designed.

    4.3   Employs procedures and techniques appropriately, efficiently and effectively.

Principle 5. The Radiologic Technologist exercises care, discretion and judgement in the practice of the profession.

    5.1   Assumes responsibility for professional decisions.

    5.2   Assesses situations and acts in the best interest of the patient.

Principle 6. The Radiologic Technologist provides the physician with pertinent information related to diagnosis and treatment management of the patient.

    6.1   Complies with the fact that diagnosis and interpretation are outside the scope of practice for the profession.

    6.2   Acts as an agent to obtain medical information through observation and communication to aid the physician in diagnosis and treatment management.

Principle 7. The Radiologic Technologist is responsible for protecting the patient, self and others from unnecessary radiation.

    7.1   Performs service with competence and expertise.

    7.2   Utilizes equipment and accessories to limit radiation to the affected area of the patient.

    7.3   Employs techniques and procedures to minimize radiation exposure to self and other members of the health care team.

Principle 8. The Radiologic Technologist practices ethical conduct befitting the profession.

    8.1   Protects the patient's right to quality radiologic technology care.

    8.2   Provides the public with information related to the profession and its functions.

    8.3   Supports the profession by maintaining and upgrading professional standards.

Code of Ethics for the Profession of Radiologic Technology—cont'd

Principle 9. The Radiologic Technologist respects confidences entrusted in the course of professional practice.

    9.1   Protects the patient's right to privacy.

    9.2   Keeps confidential, information relating to patients, colleagues and associates.

    9.3   Reveals confidential information only as required by law or to protect the welfare of the individual or the community.

Principle 10. The Radiologic Technologist recognizes that continuing education is vital to maintaining and advancing the profession.

    10.1   Participates as a student in learning activities appropriate to specific areas of responsibility as well as to the Scope of Practice.

    10.2   Shares knowledge with colleagues.

    10.3   Investigates new and innovative aspects of professional practice.

Developed by The American Society of Radiologic Technologists, June 1984.

Principle 1 is a broad, general statement that deals with "professional conduct," a dynamic concept that changes as our culture changes and is difficult to define precisely. No ideal list of acceptable behaviors exists that one can follow to guarantee that one's conduct is compatible with the dignity of the profession. Some believe that a list of rigid rules is essential. Others tend to use guidelines that are so general that they seem to represent no standards at all. Our biases regarding professional conduct are evident throughout this text and generally fall between these two extremes. We believe that a genuine commitment to serving the patient's needs, as well as those of the employer, is best achieved by taking personal responsibility for actions and by maintaining attitudes that are honest, diligent, and positive. The well-informed radiographer who approaches the profession with a truly positive intent will usually "do the right thing." Real professional integrity frees us from rigid rules but often demands that we make difficult choices. For those who fail to approach their profession with commitment, no list of rules will serve to ensure the desired outcome.

Principles 2 and 10 involve the radiographer's responsibility for continuing education and professional participation. Professional radiographers place a priority on the acquisition of additional skills and regularly expand their knowledge. Radiographers who are content with the status quo quickly find that the profession marches on without them. Standard practice changes rapidly, and today's knowledge will soon be out of date. Textbooks often contain information that is valid when the manuscript is completed but outdated by the time the book is published. Formal and informal continuing education also helps us to maintain interest in our work and to avoid the boredom and routine that are detrimental to emotional health.

In the area of professional growth, radiographers working together can accomplish much more than they can individually. To this effect, the ASRT was established in 1926. The ASRT has affiliate societies in each of the 50 states and in the Commonwealth of Puerto Rico, as well as many district groups within the state societies. These groups provide an opportunity for radiographers to become acquainted, share problems and ideas, hear speakers, present papers, and show scientific exhibits of their work. The national society and most state affiliate organizations publish journals of scientific articles and other information of interest to radiographers. Membership in these professional groups gives the radiographer an opportunity to aid in the profession's growth. Opportunities also are available to develop leadership skills through chairing committees, holding office, and participating in business and educational sessions.

The importance of scientific contribution should not be neglected. Radiographers often respond to problems or new situations by developing new methods of performing their work. Many of these ideas can be of assistance to others. All radiographers owe a large debt to those who have shared ideas to advance the art and science of radiography. We can acknowledge these gifts and receive recognition and a sense of belonging through our own contributions to the body of knowledge that is the basis of our profession (Figs. 1-4 and 1-5).

Principle 3 requires radiographers to put aside all personal prejudice and emotional bias in the process of rendering professional services. This is more difficult than it may appear at first. Most of us can easily identify prejudice in others, but our own biases or judgments are beyond our awareness or are seen by us as being fully justified or "only common sense." All of us have some natural preferences that may result in discriminatory treatment if we are not fully aware of them. With what patients do you feel most comfortable? Men? Women? Those of your own race? Those over 16? Under 30? Under 65? Middle class? Once we identify those areas in human relationships where we are most at ease, it becomes apparent that we are less at ease in some situations or would prefer to avoid them altogether. It is instructive to pay attention to how we deal with patients who are outside our "comfort zone." Sometimes we tend

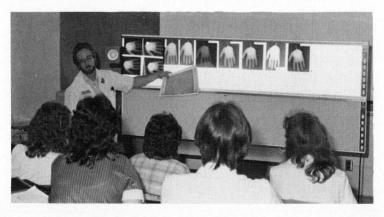

Fig. 1-4. Professional organizations help radiographers learn from one another.

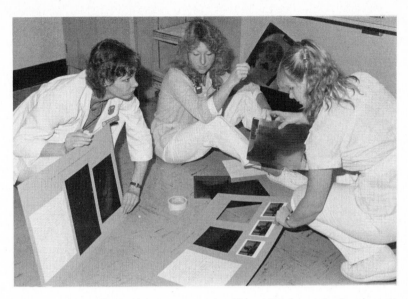

Fig. 1-5. Student radiographers prepare scientific exhibit for professional meeting.

to act more friendly or solicitous to cover up feelings. At other times we may remain aloof or may hurry. Feigned concern or pretended interest is never the same as the real thing. Faithfulness to the spirit of Principle 3 requires a high degree of self-awareness and presents a serious professional challenge to the radiographer.

Principle 4 requires that radiographers adhere to established scientific principles in the course of their work. This is necessary for the patient's safety and the profession's advancement. Since established principles change as scientific knowledge progresses, radiographers must make a consistent effort to stay current with the advancement of science as it applies to their profession. (See also Principle 10.)

Principle 5 deals with the question of professional responsibility. It implies that radiographers are truly professional because they are sufficiently educated and experienced to be capable of independent discretion and judgment. Within the scope of their professional activity, they are expected to be both capable of making decisions and accountable for the decisions they make. A very important aspect of assuming this responsibility is an awareness and an acceptance of one's limitations. Although responsibilities may vary with the working environment, regular duties should be specified in job descriptions. It is in no one's best interest to perform tasks without adequate knowledge or to undertake a responsibility without adequate qualification. This principle also holds the radiographer accountable for errors committed under the orders of another person, if the responsible radiographer knew, *or should have known*, that the order was in error.

Principle 6 specifically forbids the radiographer to diagnose; that is, the radiographer is not permitted to render a professional opinion as to the diagnosis of a patient's illness or injury. Diagnosis is defined as the act of discriminating between diseases and distinguishing them by their characteristic symptoms, or scientific discrimination between similar or related conditions for the purpose of accurate classification.

This does not mean that the radiographer should never attempt to assess a patient's condition, nor does it imply that the radiographer should be uninterested or uninformed regarding pathology or disease processes. On the contrary, the radiographer must be alert to all pertinent information that may aid in diagnosis or patient management and report this to the physician (see also Chapter 4). However, the radiographer's education does not provide the comprehensive background necessary for diagnosis. This responsibility, which includes the diagnostic interpretation of radiographs and other diagnostic images, lies solely with the physician.

Principle 7 requires that the radiographer make *every effort* to protect *all* patients from unnecessary radiation. Although the technical aspects of radiation protection are beyond the scope of this text, some practical guidelines are provided in Appendix D. The ethical implications of this issue are very important. When a radiographer violates this principle, there is no telltale evidence. The negative consequences of other breaches of ethics might be immediate, but the latent and genetic effects of unnecessary radiation to patients may not be apparent for 10 to 20 years or even for several generations. Making every effort to protect the patient—even when the patient is difficult to handle, even when you have been awakened for an emergency in the middle of the night, even when you are really in a hurry, and even when no one is watching—requires both good habits and a strong ethical commitment to radiation protection.

Principle 8 defines the radiographer's responsibility with respect to patient rights (see p. 15 and Appendix A). It also establishes the radiographer's relationship to the public regarding misinformation and misrepresentation. Radiographers are seen to by the public as experts on both radiation and health, and they should be aware of the responsibility that this image imposes. A careless or misleading statement may spread through the lay community as the official word of a respected authority. Radiographers can take several steps to fulfill the intent of this principle:

1. Be well informed and up-to-date.
2. Take pride in professional status but carefully avoid misrepresenting knowledge, position, or authority.
3. Say "I don't know" when this is the case, and resist the temptation to bluff.
4. Cooperate with professional organizations in providing accurate information about matters of professional interest and concern.

Principle 9 relates to the confidentiality of information in a health care setting, which is one of the cardinal concepts in all codes of ethics relating to health care. The confidentiality of conversations between patients and their physicians is considered so important that, along with communications to lawyers and the clergy, it is protected by "legal privilege." This means that the professional cannot be required to divulge such information, even when to do so might be of material value in a court of law. The information provided to a radiographer is *not* legally privileged, but radiographers are often privy to conversations between patients and their physicians, as well as to confidential information contained in patient charts. They often witness circumstances in which patients are unable to preserve their dignity and may behave in ways that might cause them shame or embarrassment if known to friends or family. Many patients do not want it known that they are ill or have been hospitalized. Some may wish to keep their diagnosis confidential. Information that may seem of no consequence to you may constitute a very sensitive issue for the patient. Any breach of confidence, even if no names are mentioned, may rightly be interpreted by others as an indication that the radiographer does not respect professional confidence. Betrayals of confidence cause individuals to lose faith in the health care team and may result in their hesitation to reveal facts essential to their care.

The patient's right to confidentiality is not violated by appropriate communications among health care workers when the information is pertinent to the patient's care. It is justifiably assumed in such a case that the transfer of information is for the patient's benefit and that all personnel involved are bound by the ethics regarding confidentiality. Appropriate communications are those directed privately to those who have need of the information. Conversations about patients must never be held in public areas such as waiting rooms, elevators, or cafeterias.

The ethics of patient-staff communication also require the exercise of sound judgment and restraint to avoid exposing to patients the radiographer's personal concerns or the problems of the hospital staff. Using the patient as a sounding board for complaints or gossip is inexcusable.

Patient rights

A major aspect of ethical concern for radiographers is to protect patient rights at all times. Increasing emphasis is being placed on consumer advocacy in our society, and this trend is especially significant in the field of health care. An example of a patient's rights statement is on p. 16. A more comprehensive statement is found in Appendix A. Several of these concepts are especially pertinent to the work of radiographers.

Foremost is the right to considerate and respectful care. This statement is self-explanatory and applies to every patient, regardless of current status.

The patient also has a right to information, but this does *not* place an obligation on the radiographer to provide any and all information that may be requested. Radiographers must be prepared to offer explanations of radiographic procedures and to identify themselves and the radiologists. Questions regarding diagnosis, treatment, and other aspects of care should be referred to the physician.

Although patient consent to routine procedures is given on admission and is implied by the continued acceptance of hospital care, informed consent is necessary for any procedure that is considered experimental or that involves substantial risk. In the radiology department, certain procedures, such as arteriograms, require that the patient receive an explanation of both the procedure

A Patient's Bill of Rights

1. The patient has the right to considerate and respectful care.

2. The patient has the right to obtain from his physician complete current information concerning his diagnosis, treatment, and prognosis in terms the patient can be reasonably expected to understand. When it is not medically advisable to give such information to the patient, the information should be made available to an appropriate person in his behalf. He has the right to know, by name, the physician responsible for his care.

3. The patient has the right to receive from his physician information necessary to give informed consent prior to the start of any procedure and/or treatment. Except in emergencies, such information for informed consent should include, but not necessarily be limited to, the specific procedure and/or treatment, the medically significant risks involved, and the probable duration of incapacitation. Where medically significant alternatives for care or treatment exist, or when the patient requests information concerning medical alternatives, the patient has the right to such information. The patient also has the right to know the name of the person responsible for the procedures and/or treatment.

4. The patient has the right to refuse treatment to the extent permitted by law and to be informed of the medical consequences of his action.

5. The patient has the right to every consideration of his privacy concerning his own medical care program. Case discussion, consultation, examination, and treatment are confidential and should be conducted discreetly. Those not directly involved in his care must have the permission of the patient to be present.

6. The patient has the right to expect that all communications and records pertaining to his care should be treated as confidential.

7. The patient has the right to expect that within its capacity a hospital must make reasonable response to the request of a patient for services. The hospital must provide evaluation, service, and/or referral as indicated by the urgency of the case. When medically permissible, a patient may be transferred to another facility only after he has received complete information and explanation concerning the needs for and alternatives to such a transfer. The institution to which the patient is to be transferred must first have accepted the patient for transfer.

8. The patient has the right to obtain information as to any relationship of his hospital to other health care and educational institutions insofar as his care is concerned. The patient has the right to obtain information as to the existence of any professional relationships among individuals, by name, who are treating him.

9. The patient has the right to be advised if the hospital proposes to engage in or perform human experimentation affecting his care or treatment. The patient has the right to refuse to participate in such research projects.

10. The patient has the right to expect reasonable continuity of care. He has the right to know in advance what appointment times and physicians are available and where. The patient has the right to expect that the hospital will provide a mechanism whereby he is informed by his physician or a delegate of the physician of the patient's continuing health care requirements following discharge.

11. The patient has the right to examine and receive an explanation of his bill, regardless of source of payment.

12. The patient has the right to know what hospital rules and regulations apply to his conduct as a patient.

Reprinted with the permission of the American Hospital Association. Copyright 1975.

and the potential risk and sign a consent form. For some patients, providing information and obtaining consent is the physician's duty, but for patients undergoing most routine procedures, a staff member provides the necessary form and explanation.

When it is your duty to obtain informed consent, be sure that you are prepared with a full understanding of the procedure and its risks so that you can give an adequate explanation to the patient and answer any questions. If the patient asks a question that you are not prepared for, seek the correct answer before continuing. An improper response may invalidate the consent. The legal implications of informed consent cannot be overemphasized. Successful litigation has been based on lack of compliance with the following guidelines:

1. Patients must receive a full explanation of the procedure and its risks and sign the consent form *before* being sedated or anesthetized.
2. A patient must be competent in order to sign an informed consent.
3. Only parents or legal guardians may sign for a minor.
4. Only a legal guardian may sign for a mentally incompetent patient.
5. Consent forms must be completed before being signed. Patients should never be asked to sign a blank form or a form with blank spaces "to be filled in later."
6. Only the physician named on the consent form may perform the procedure. Consent is not transferable from one physician to another, even an associate.
7. Any condition stated on the form must be met. For example, if the form states that a family member will be present during the procedure, the consent is not valid if the family member is not in attendance.

A typical consent form is reproduced in Appendix B. It is the radiographer's responsibility to be aware of which procedures require written consent and to check the chart to be certain that these forms are in order before proceeding with the examination.

The right to refuse treatment also implies the right to refuse examination. If a patient chooses to exercise this right, the radiographer *must not* proceed with the study. Note that signing an informed consent does not invalidate the patient's right to refuse treatment once the procedure has begun. Consent may be revoked at any time during the procedure. If this occurs, take time to explore the reason why the patient is unwilling to continue. This may be a response to a temporary discomfort and not an objection to the procedure itself. If the patient still refuses to complete the procedure, comply gracefully and allow the patient to leave or return to the nursing service. The attending physician must be notified.

The right of privacy implies that the patient's modesty will be respected and that every effort will be made to assist the patient in maintaining a sense of personal dignity. The radiographer must remember that many common procedures (e.g., enemas) threaten the patient's modesty and dignity; patients are likely to be much more sensitive in these situations than the health care workers, for whom the procedures are an everyday occurrence.

Somewhat related to this right is the generally accepted practice to ensure that a patient and a physician or other health care worker of opposite sexes are not left alone together in a setting that requires undraping of the patient or examination of the genitalia or female breasts. A "chaperone," preferably of the same sex as the patient, should be present if at all possible. The objective of the practice is not to prevent the health professional from violating ethical principles, although this may be a consideration. The main purpose is to ease the patient's mind if he or she fears such an encounter and to provide a witness in case the patient later claims to have been assaulted or touched in an unprofessional manner. Many institutions have policies that apply in these situations, and many physicians prefer to be chaperoned, even when no such policy exists. The radiographer should be aware of the institution's policies and sensitive to other's needs in this regard.

Note that students and others not required for a procedure must have the patient's permission to be present. The taking of photographs, other than for the sole purpose of the patient's care, also requires consent.

The right of privacy also includes the expectation of confidentiality, discussed earlier in this chapter.

Death with dignity.   Although not mentioned in the Patient's Bill of Rights, considerable public attention has been given in recent years to the patient's right to die. This can present a serious ethical conflict between health care workers' commitment to do everything possible to preserve and prolong life and the patient's right to die with dignity. Recently the media have focused much attention on the controversial subject of euthanasia, or mercy killing. In the United States, euthanasia is still considered a crime, regardless of the circumstances. Resuscitation of patients for whom there is a reasonable expectation of recovery is definitely considered to be medically and ethically correct. A vast gray area lies between these two situations, however, which has become an issue since modern technology has made it possible to sustain life indefinitely by providing artificial life support to persons who would otherwise not survive. Heroic measures may only serve to prolong the patient's suffering at great cost to the family and the public.

When the patient's condition is terminal and when the physician and the patient agree (or the patient's family, if the patient is incompetent), a "no-code" or "do not resuscitate" (DNR) order may be written. This means that if death is imminent, no effort at resuscitation is to be attempted. When a no-code order is instituted, a notation is placed in the patient's chart so that all who care for the patient will be aware of the order.

Many older patients choose to sign a *living will,* which states that in the event of an illness or accident, they do not wish life-sustaining measures if they have little or no chance of resuming a meaningful quality of life. Copies of this "will" are usually given to the family physician and an attorney or family member.

Another way for individuals to participate in long-term decision making about their health care is to initiate a *power of attorney for health care.* This action enables a trusted person to act on the patient's behalf if and when the patient is unable to act. The designated person should be aware of the patient's wishes to make appropriate decisions. This person is empowered to sign a valid informed consent form.

Self-care

A radiographer who is not healthy is not a good health role model and cannot function effectively for both physical and psychological reasons. To help others, we must first meet our own physical and mental needs. Certain needs are common to everyone and can be listed and ranked in importance (Fig. 1-6). Any unmet need imposes stress and prevents us from achieving our optimum state of well-being.

Needs on the most elemental level are foremost until they are adequately satisfied. As satisfaction occurs on one level, the needs of the next higher level occupy the individual's attention. Self-actualization is the state in which a person welcomes tension and effort as a stimulus to creativity and self-expression. Your need for esteem and self-actualization may be the reason you are a student in this program. Constructively meeting our needs for well-being, knowledge, and self-esteem enables us to function more fully, free from self-preoccupation at those times when the patient requires full attention.

Since many patients have a lowered resistance that makes them especially vulnerable to infection, the radiographer who is ill should stay at home. However, since the team is counting on all members being there when scheduled, it is even better to prevent the onset of illness. The serious disturbances we are all subject to occasionally, such as grief or undue worry, should be considered as illnesses and treated as such. One should stay at home and rest or otherwise deal with such problems. One who is anxious cannot properly fulfill responsibilities.

The practice of good nutrition and exercise habits may sound trite but pays off in less time lost from work and an increased sense of well-being. Knowledge and practice of the principles of body mechanics (see Chapter 3) help one avoid the types of injuries that most frequently result from lifting and moving patients or equipment.

Preventive health measures are equally important. For example, hospitals are required to offer employees hepatitis B vaccine, but you are responsible for taking advantage of this important protection. The universal precautions discussed in Chapter 5 have been developed to help prevent transmission of blood-borne diseases from patient to patient and from patient to you. Such precautions are completely useless unless you understand and use the principles involved. Minimizing the risk of disease in a health care setting depends on your willingness

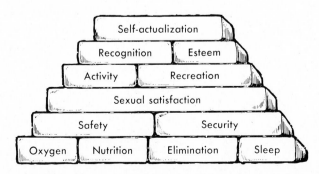

Fig. 1-6. Hierarchy of human needs.

to learn and use the information offered to you.

Radiation exposure over the course of a career can have serious health consequences if proper precautions are not observed. Your curriculum will include an extensive study of radiation protection. Adhering to radiation safety practices is another important aspect of self-care.

Care of supplies and equipment

Ethical conduct applies to the care of objects as well as people. Hospitals stock tremendous quantities of supplies to function effectively. In such an environment, one can easily assume that free access implies free use. In truth, however, someone must pay the bill. To the purchase price of each inventory item one must add on an overhead factor that may be two or three times the item's basic value. For example, to the cost of a film that is accidentally exposed one must add the proportional cost in work hours of the stock clerk, receiving clerk, purchasing agent, and accountant, as well as the administrators who supervise these employees. One must also consider overhead costs for shipping and storage.

Medical equipment is expensive, and proper care is required to ensure that its value is preserved and that it is available for use when needed. The misuse of equipment or supplies or their diversion for personal use wastes funds and increases health care costs. The radiographer who avoids such waste is demonstrating a high standard of ethical behavior.

Legal considerations

Intentional misconduct.   Personal injury lawsuits are becoming more and more common in the field of health care. They usually fall into one of two categories; *intentional misconduct* or *negligence*. The types of misconduct that occur in the hospital are assault, battery, false imprisonment, invasion of privacy, libel, and slander (defamation of character).

Assault may be defined as the *threat* of touching in an injurious way. Note that the person need not be touched in any way for assault to occur. If the patient feels threatened and is caused to believe that he or she will be touched in a harmful manner, justification may exist for a charge of assault. To avoid this, the radiographer *must* explain what is to occur and reassure the patient in any situation where the threat of harm may be an issue. Never use threats to gain the patient's cooperation; this applies to pediatric as well as adult patients.

Battery consists of an unlawful touching of a person without consent. If the patient refuses to be touched, that wish must be respected. Even the most well-intentioned touch may fall into this category if the patient has expressly forbidden it. This should not prevent the radiographer from placing a reassuring hand on the patient's shoulder, as long as the patient has not forbidden it, when there is no intent to harm or to invade the patient's privacy. On the other hand, a radiograph taken against the patient's will or on the wrong patient could be construed as battery. This emphasizes the need for consistently double checking patient identification and being certain that proper informed consent has been obtained for procedures that require it.

False imprisonment is the unjustifiable detention of a person against his or her will. This becomes an issue when the patient wishes to leave and is not allowed to do so. Inappropriate use of physical restraints may also constitute false imprisonment. Reasonable judgment must be used to decide whether restraints are necessary. Most hospitals have policies requiring restraints for patient safety, for example, using safety belts on stretchers and using side rails on hospital beds at night.

Invasion of privacy charges may result when confidentiality of information has not been maintained or when the patient's body has been improperly and unnecessarily exposed or touched. The significance of confidentiality has already been emphasized. Hospitals and their employees may be liable if they disclose confidential information obtained from a patient or contained in the medical record. If the information disclosed reflects negatively on the patient's reputation, one may also be liable for defamation of character. Liability can also result if photographs are published without a patient's permission. Protection of the patient's modesty is vitally important as well and is noted throughout this text as it pertains to specific procedures.

Libel and *slander* refer to the malicious spreading of information that results in *defamation of character* or loss of reputation. Usually, libel refers to written information, and slander is more often applied to information spread verbally. Therefore, breach of the confidentiality rules is not only unethical but also may cause the radiographer to be sued for slander.

Negligence and malpractice.   Negligence, on the other hand, refers to the neglect or omission of reasonable care or caution. The standard of reasonable care is based on the "doctrine of the reasonably prudent person." This standard requires that a person perform as any reasonable person would perform under similar circumstances. In the relationship between a professional person and a patient or client, the professional has a duty to provide reasonable care. An act of negligence in the context of such a relationship is defined as *professional negligence* or *malpractice*. The radiographer is held to the standard of care and skill of the "reasonable radiographer" in similar circumstances. You may hear the terms *gross negligence* and *contributory negligence*. Gross negligence refers to negligent acts that involve "reckless disregard for life or limb." It carries a higher degree of negligence than ordinary negligence and results in more serious penalties. Contributory negligence refers to an act of negligence in which the behavior of the injured party contributed to the injurious outcome.

Malpractice lawsuits against physicians and hospitals also are becoming increasingly common. As a result, rates for malpractice insurance coverage have soared in recent years, and this topic is a serious concern to all health professionals.

Legally, to establish a claim of malpractice, a claimant must prove to the court's satisfaction that four conditions are true: (1) the person or institution being sued had a duty to provide reasonable care to the patient; (2) the patient has sustained some loss or injury; (3) the person or institution being sued is the party responsible for the loss; and (4) the loss is attributable to negligence or improper practice. Accordingly, a patient may sustain some loss, but for the patient to collect damages, the court must be convinced that the loss has resulted from negligence in professional care or treatment. Usually a determination of negligence is based on whether or not the usual standards and procedures for the particular situation were followed in the case in question. In another case a patient may prove that someone was negligent but may not be entitled to a settlement unless it can be demonstrated that a loss has occurred as a result. Nonetheless, it is inexcusable to be complacent about negligence simply because there was "no harm done." Also, one should not be callous about loss just because accepted and established procedures were followed.

There has been much discussion concerning whether radiographers should carry malpractice insurance. Hospitals carry liability insurance, which covers negligence of employees acting in the course of their employment. Radiographers must learn the extent of provisions for malpractice coverage in their institutions. According to the legal doctrine of *respondeat superior* ("let the master respond"), the employer is liable for employees' negligent acts that occur in the course of their work. In recent years, however, the "rule of personal responsibility" has been increasingly applied. This means that *each person is liable for his or her own negligent conduct*. Under this rule the law does not allow the wrongdoer to escape responsibility, even though someone else may be legally liable as well.

Malpractice lawsuits have resulted in unfavorable judgments against radiographers as individuals. In rare cases, hospital insurers who have paid malpractice claims have successfully recovered damages from negligent employees by filing separate suits against them. Some believe these are sufficient reasons for radiographers to be protected by their own liability insurance policies. Others argue that the potential for a large insurance settlement is an incentive to sue and that if the radiographer has no means of paying a large claim, no suit will be filed. The ASRT offers professional liability coverage on a group basis, indicating that this organization thinks such coverage is important. The possibility of losing personal assets, such as one's home, may provide motivation for joining such a plan.

Lawsuits can result in conflict, expense, professional embarrassment, and loss of public confidence even when the patient is denied any award. Thus a great need exists for caution both in the interest of patient care and in the avoidance of possible malpractice claims. Research indicates that lawsuits are most likely when patients feel alienated from the people providing their care. When a trusting professional relationship is established, suits are less likely to occur. With this in mind, David Karp, Loss Prevention Manager of Medical Insurance Exchange of California, has developed the following list of the seven Cs of malpractice prevention.*

1. **Competence.** Knowing and adhering to professional standards and maintaining professional competence reduce liability exposure.
2. **Compliance.** The compliance by health professionals with policies and procedures in the medical office and hospital avoids patient injuries and litigation.

---

*The seven Cs are printed here with the permission of David Karp.

3. **Charting.** Charting completely, consistently, and objectively can be the best defense against a malpractice claim.
4. **Communication.** Patient injuries and resulting malpractice cases can be avoided by improving communications among health care professionals.
5. **Confidentiality.** Protecting the confidentiality of medical information is a legal and ethical responsibility of health professionals.
6. **Courtesy.** A courteous attitude and demeanor can improve patient rapport and lessen the likelihood of lawsuits.
7. **Carefulness.** Personal injuries on the premises which lead to lawsuits can occur unexpectedly (See Chapter 3).

Proper patient identification, accuracy in medication administration, and compliance with patient safety requirements are positive steps the radiographer can take to avoid malpractice suits. Harm may result from contrast media administered when proper precautions are not observed or when reactions are not immediately identified and appropriately treated. Poor radiographs pose a potential for misdiagnosis that may have serious consequences for both patient and radiographer. Potential for harmful error is often greatest in stressful situations. Appropriate responses in an emergency ensure the least possible risk. You must understand and accept that an appropriate response depends on your level of experience and education. Do not hesitate to ask questions and receive help when needed.

The radiographer can also protect the institution and the patient by reporting illegal or unethical professional activities to the proper authorities. In such a situation the radiographer must take care to be neither too zealous nor too hesitant. A simple, written statement that includes the facts (dates, times, names, places) but avoids conclusions, speculations, or judgments should be prepared and submitted to the appropriate person, probably one's immediate supervisor, unless he or she was involved in the incident. One should write down the facts of such an occurrence as soon as possible after observing them. The supervisor receiving such a report is responsible for seeing that it is given to the proper authority, who must then follow up by investigating. A single report may not produce change, but it may add strength to other reports or lead to increased supervision where needed.

CONCLUSION

The health care team consists of a large group of people with varied skills and responsibilities. It is organized to form a chain of command that is effective in providing the best possible patient care. The radiographer is an important member of this team with significant responsibilities to patients and to the team. To meet these responsibilities, radiographers must first provide for their own physical and emotional health.

Professional groups offer opportunities for continuing education and professional growth and also establish standards for ethical behavior. Ethical and professional behavior is essential to good patient care. Such conduct safeguards patient rights and reduces the likelihood of medicolegal difficulties.

Study questions

1. List four ways in which adherence to the ASRT Code of Ethics might help a radiographer to avoid an accusation of malpractice.
2. Using "A Patient's Bill of Rights" from this chapter, identify those patient rights for which a radiographer may have direct responsibility.
3. Diagram the structure that forms the "chain of command" in the radiology department at your clinical facility.

Attitudes and Communication in Patient Care

Vocabulary list

1. acute
2. aggressive
3. ambulatory
4. aphasia
5. assertive
6. autonomy
7. cholecystography
8. chronic
9. degenerative
10. dermatitis
11. diarrhea
12. empathy
13. hypertension
14. regimen
15. resuscitation

PROFESSIONAL ATTITUDES

Health-illness continuum

The delivery of health care can be viewed in many ways. *Crisis intervention* is an approach in which the patient or client seeks help only when unable to manage alone. As soon as the emergency or inability to manage has passed, the former pattern of life is resumed. The *health maintenance* or *preventive* health system, on the other hand, attempts to promote well-being and avoid the need for intensive medical intervention. It encourages better nutrition, exercise, and hygiene habits. Potential health problems are identified before they manifest as illness. Early illnesses are treated before they become chronic or life-threatening.

These two approaches are not mutually exclusive, since each deals with different stages on a line that could be drawn from optimum health to fatal illness. Such a line is referred to as the *health-illness continuum*. An example of such a continuum is a healthy patient required to obtain a chest radiograph for employment purposes or to establish baseline data for a complete health survey. On the other end of the spectrum, you could encounter a critical patient whose study may provide life-saving data or a terminal patient whose examination may be primarily for the benefit of research. Since patients in the radiology department may fall anywhere along this health-illness continuum, you must be both empathetic and flexible in your approach to such varying needs. As health care becomes more complex and more expensive, any measures you can take to promote health will shorten hospital stays and prevent duplication of services. This increases cost-effectiveness and patient satisfaction as well.

Developing professional attitudes

Health is a state of physical, mental, and social well-being, and to be healthy implies that one is capable of promoting health. Health professionals are responsible for their own well-being and also serve as health role models for their patients. Members of the health team must take care not to project the attitude, "Do as I say, not as I do," and thus undermine their credibility in the eyes of the very people they most want to help.

Most students enter radiography because it is a caring, helping profession. The desire to help is not enough. The demands of clinical practice often tend to overshadow humanitarian considerations. The patient's needs may be overlooked in the stress of coping with highly technical material unless you make a conscious effort to learn, from the beginning, to handle both at once.

Your work will be most satisfying to you when your contributions and the personal contacts they involve are genuine and sincere. When you do things because you *want* to do them and you *enjoy* doing them, you will do them well. Therefore, begin with a commitment to quality in both performance and relationships, and seek opportunities to express your commitment in all you do.

Dealing effectively with clinical situations involves several abilities. One is the ability to show *empathy*, a sensitivity to the needs of others that allows you to meet those needs constructively, rather than merely sympathizing, or reacting to their distress. Understanding and compassion are accompanied by an objective detachment that enables you to provide an appropriate response. For example, you could express sympathy for the victim of a tragic accident by crying or by smothering him with expressions of pity. On the other hand, an expression of empathy would show concern and tenderness while providing the films that would aid in rapid diagnosis and treatment.

It is also very useful to cultivate the ability to be *assertive*. This does not imply that you need to be *aggressive*. Expressions of aggression involve anger or hostility, whereas assertion is the calm, firm expression of feelings or opinions. As students you have the right to be assertive when you require assistance in a patient care situation that is beyond your ability. Employers may be assertive in requiring employees to maintain the level of competence required by their job descriptions. In dealing with patients who are reluctant to cooperate, pleasant assertiveness is the attitude that is most productive in obtaining compliance.

A focus on patient needs will enable you to respond calmly and assertively when a patient's actions are inappropriate. It may seem strange or frightening to you that some individuals respond to stress or anxiety by becoming hostile or even threatening. These are often people whose coping mechanism depends on being in control or "on top of" the situation. Preserving an extremely calm, objective attitude is most effective in dealing with such patients. Overt expressions of sexuality by patients are encountered very infrequently. Such events are usually a reflection of anxiety by patients who no longer feel functional as sexual human beings because of their current physical status. With this in mind, you can be less judgmental about specific behaviors and face the patient directly. You can refuse to accept the behavior while continuing to reassure and care for the patient.

A focus on patient needs is also helpful when coping with other concerns often expressed by beginning students, such as, "What shall I do if the patient vomits? I just know I'll get sick, too!" or "I faint at the sight of blood." As you gain experience in your education, you will learn to deal with the emergency first and let your knees shake later. The effort to project a calm, reassuring attitude to the patient will be your best reinforcement.

Dealing with dying and death

The terminally ill patient is in an emotional state of grieving. This process is experienced by anyone who suffers serious loss and is typical of patients who become handicapped or disfigured. Grief is also experienced by the families of grieving patients and of those who have died.

Dr. Elisabeth Kübler-Ross has studied and written extensively on the subject of death and dying over the past 25 years. Her work has greatly changed the way members of the helping professions view the dying process and assist those who are terminally ill. She points out that grief is an emotional readjustment to a new way of experiencing life and cannot be accomplished all at once. She identifies five phases of the grieving process:

1. **Denial.** At this stage the grieving person refuses to accept the truth and usually refuses to discuss the possibility of loss or death.
2. **Anger.** As denial is overcome, the patient experiences the frustration of helplessness and a feeling of outrage at the apparent injustice of the loss. Rage may be vented on family, friends, and health care workers. This may be beyond the patient's control.

3. **Bargaining.** At this stage the patient seems to be attempting to earn forgiveness or mitigation of the loss by being "very good." Patients in this phase of grief are conscientious about following physicians' orders, are considerate of others, and seldom complain, even when suffering.
4. **Depression.** The depressed patient is acquiescent, quiet, and withdrawn and may cry easily.
5. **Acceptance.** At the conclusion of the grieving process the patient accepts the loss or impending death and deals with life and relationships on a more realistic, day-to-day basis. Patients who accept their loss are comfortable talking about it and generally display attitudes that are appropriate to their immediate circumstances.

Although the grieving process is facilitated by supportive acceptance of the patient at each stage of grief, the time required to pass from one phase to the next varies with individuals and cannot be hurried.

In dealing with the grieving patient, the radiographer may be presented with statements or questions that require a sensitive response. The patient may say, "I wish it was all over," "How long do you think I have to live?" or "Don't you think I'm much better today?" when there has been no change. In such circumstances the radiographer may feel a strong tendency to respond with the language of denial. A typical denial statement might be, "Don't talk like that; you're going to be fine." Such responses tend to block communication and may be insulting to the patient who has long since passed the phase of denial. One should remember that the patient is not necessarily seeking a direct response. What is needed is a friendly, supportive listener. Rephrasing the patient's remark encourages the patient to talk and conveys a message of acceptance. Examples of such responses to the previous remarks might be, "You're feeling tired of living," "You'd like to know how long you have to live," or "You're feeling better today?" Do not be afraid to be involved or to show that you care. Be lavish with touch and comfort measures.

In an acute care hospital, despite the most sophisticated emergency resuscitation systems, patients sometimes die. The medical and nursing staffs have developed definite procedures to follow in the case of death, and these responsibilities do not normally include the radiographer. The physician notifies the family while the nursing staff prepares the body for transport to the morgue. Your role might be to provide support for the family while awaiting word from the physician. If so, do not volunteer information or discuss the staff's actions. Your observations and opinions must not be discussed at this time. When the family reaches the anger phase of their grieving process, they may want to place blame for an unavoidable death. Spontaneous comments made under stress are sometimes quoted by families in court actions to support accusations of malpractice. If you have any question about the appropriateness of the staff's actions surrounding a patient death, this should be evaluated later, in private, with your supervisor.

When a patient dies, the excitement and bustle of resuscitation procedures may carry you through the acute event. The period that follows is important to your mental health. Talk about your feelings with a supportive person. Health professionals often see themselves as rescuers, and these unrealistic expectations may lead to feelings of inadequacy and depression when a patient dies. Do not be afraid to cry. All human beings are unique, and the death of any one of us diminishes humankind. Few professionals are totally comfortable in the presence of death. Most of us find it difficult to face our own mortality and eventual death with objectivity, but those who work in an acute care setting must learn to accept death as yet another aspect of living. We strongly urge you to expand your awareness by reading and discussing this sensitive subject. (See Chapter 1 regarding the patient's right to die and no-code orders.)

PRINCIPLES OF COMMUNICATION

Nonverbal communication

Implied in any list of basic human needs is the need to communicate effectively with each other. How do we accomplish this? Language is the primary means, but we also use much nonverbal behavior to let others know how we feel about them. Literature provides us with the interpretation of many nonverbal behaviors. Everyone can recognize some of the more common ones. We usually perceive frowns or pursed lips as disapproval. Refusal to look directly into an individual's face while speaking conveys avoidance or rejection, and clenched teeth or fists suggest anger. With what other common nonverbal behaviors are you familiar? (See Fig. 2-1.)

Touch is a means of communication, too. An abrupt or gingerly touch may be seen as distaste or reluctance to care for the individual. A positive touch is firm but gentle (Fig. 2-2) and reassures the patient that you are both capable and caring. Everyone we meet receives some impression of who we are. What

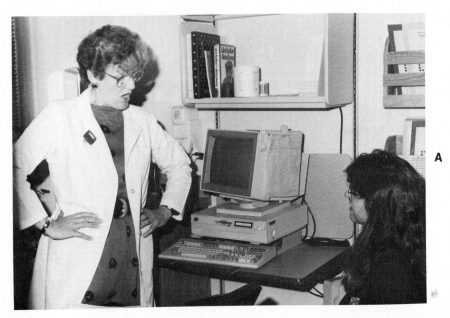

A

Fig. 2-1. A, What do you think is being communicated?

Continued.

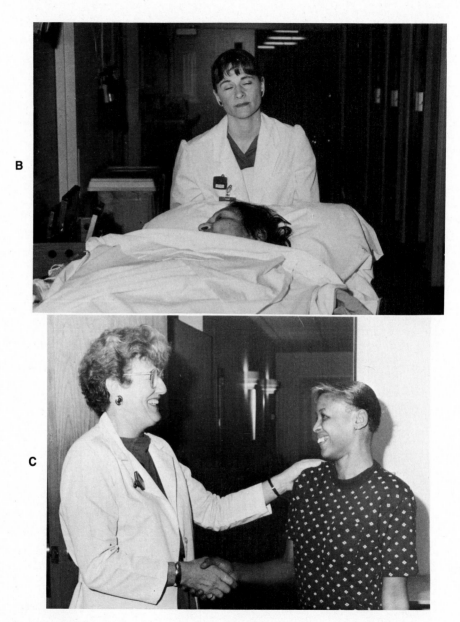

Fig. 2-1, cont'd.   B, Appearances can be deceiving. Is this radiographer exasperated or merely tired? **C,** Genuine reassurance without words.

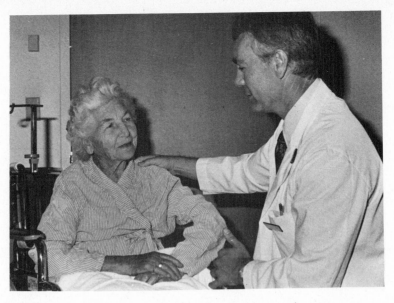

Fig. 2-2. Positive touch is firm but gentle.

does your appearance tell your patients about you? Appearance is another means of communicating how we feel about our work and our patients. The best radiographers love their work and their patients. They treat patients with the same concern that they would appreciate if they were ill. They realize that some people are rigid and intolerant, especially when feeling anxious. Such patients will place their confidence in the radiographer only if their expectations of a professional person are being met. Uniforms are worn by radiographers to present a simple, neat appearance. They are washable and plain to make them easy to keep clean. They should fit comfortably and be worn with simple, appropriate accessories. Although fads and fashions change over time, a professional image will continue to be conservative.

The appearance of the examining room is equally important. An untidy, cluttered room does not show respect for patients. It suggests that personnel may be too pressured or too uncaring to answer questions or provide reassurance (Fig. 2-3).

Listening skills

How do you feel when you are interrupted or when the listener looks out the window while you attempt to make your point? Are you irritated when others "put words in your mouth" or change the subject without responding to what you have just said? Good communication is a two-way street. A good listener does more than wait his or her turn to speak. Listening skill involves the ability to focus on the speaker, maintain eye contact, and respond to what has been said.

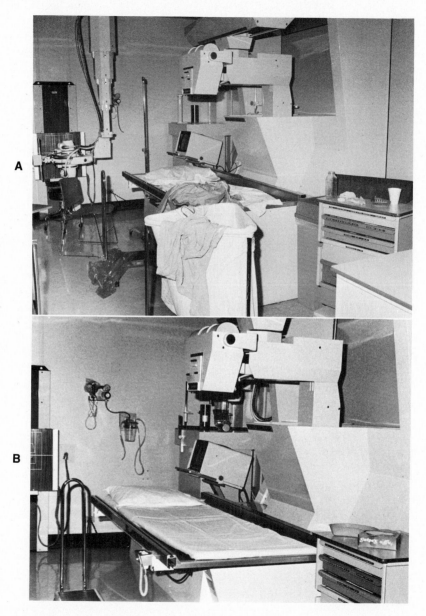

Fig. 2-3.   Appearance of a room affects a patient's attitude toward care. **A,** What does this room communicate to you? **B,** A clean room inspires confidence.

Validation of communication

Being a good communicator implies the ability to use language and content appropriate to your listeners and to validate whether you have been understood. An informal response such as a smile, nod, or brief "OK" may be a satisfactory acknowledgment in a social situation, but when essential information is being presented, the response must be one that reflects clear understanding. This is particularly true with all instructions that involve your professional activities. As a listener, you can be sure that you have understood the message by reflecting the elements of the speaker's statement in your response:

> *Speaker:* "Give Mrs. Johnson 50 ml of Isovue 300, and take the first film at 60 seconds."
>
> *Listener:* "Mrs. Johnson gets 50 ml of Isovue 300, and I'll take the first film at 60 seconds."
>
> *Speaker:* "Right."

In this communication the speaker's instruction is complete. The listener's response reflects complete understanding, and that understanding is validated.

When the speaker receives an incomplete response, the situation changes:

> *Speaker:* Give Mrs. Johnson 50 ml Isovue 100, and take the first film at 3 minutes.
>
> *Listener:* OK. (Turns to leave.)

At this point the speaker cannot be certain of having been understood, so the conversation must be continued:

> *Speaker:* "Wait, tell me what you're going to do."
>
> *Listener:* I'll give Mrs. Johnson 50 ml of Isovue and take the first film at 3 minutes."
>
> *Speaker:* "What strength Isovue?"
>
> *Listener:* "Isovue 300."
>
> *Speaker:* "No, Isovue 100 this time."
>
> *Listener:* "Oh, OK; 50 ml of Isovue 100."
>
> *Speaker:* "Right."

When presented with an incomplete message, the listener's responsibility is to obtain *clarification:*

> *Speaker:* "Give her 50 ml of Isovue."
>
> *Listener:* "That's 50 ml of Isovue 300 for Mrs. Johnson and the first film at 60 seconds as usual?"
>
> *Speaker:* "Right."

If the listener's assumption was incorrect, the speaker must then state the intended message more accurately:

> *Speaker:* "No, no. Mrs. Johnson should have 50 ml of Isovue 100 because of her decreased renal function, then start the filming at 3 minutes for the same reason."
>
> *Listener:* "OK; 50 ml of Isovue 100 and film at 3 minutes."
>
> *Speaker:* "Right."

In this case the speaker did not provide some essential information. Both parties might have assumed that they were referring to the same patient and that the usual dose of Isovue and routine time would be used for the examination. When these points are not clear, the potential for error is greater.

The lesson for both speakers and listeners is that messages must be clear and complete and that understanding must be *validated* or confirmed. Without validation, neither party can proceed with the assurance of clear understanding.

Communication under stress

Any situation that disturbs our everyday activities imposes stress. Most health care involves some stress, and the hospital environment often proves stressful to patients, families, and health care workers. This is especially true in crisis situations when speed is a factor or when disagreement exists about what should be done.

Stress interferes with our ability to process information accurately or appropriately. We have all read newspaper accounts about victims of a house fire who fled with the closest object, such as the rubber plant, rather than important papers or possessions. In a stressful situation, accurate communication can be difficult. The principles of communication already discussed are always important, but these additional suggestions can improve your effectiveness in a crisis:

1. Lower your voice and speak slowly and clearly when a situation is very emotional.
2. Be nonjudgmental in both verbal and nonverbal communication. Do not allow an upset individual's inappropriate actions or speech to goad you into a similar response.
3. When you are uncertain whether the listener has understood you, request an answer, for example, "Did you read the consent form? What did it say?"

Extremely stressful situations may evoke responses that are hostile or even violent. If you express distaste or hostility, this can escalate the level of tension. Occasionally a patient who is recovering consciousness will become combative, or an elderly patient who is disoriented may threaten violent action. However, most potentially violent situations occur in the emergency room, such as a patient involved in a motor vehicle accident that might have been caused by drunk driving and who has been brought in by the police for examination or care or a group of individuals brought in following an unresolved fight. The essential points to remember in such situations are:

1. Do not attempt to cope alone. Ask for help before the problem escalates, and leave the room if physical violence is threatened.
2. Be pleasantly firm while explaining that your role is to provide health care only.
3. Never let a combative individual get between you and the door.
4. Review with your supervisor and co-workers how to handle such situations before they arise.

COMMUNICATION WITH PATIENTS

Addressing the patient

The first contact with a patient is usually an introduction. In many social situations today, given names are used as soon as introductions are made. Although this may project an air of friendliness and informality, it also poses certain problems. As mentioned earlier, the hospital environment induces varying amounts of stress, and in many people this is reflected as a strong feeling of helplessness or loss of autonomy. Patients are told where and when to lie down, what to eat, when to take medications, and so on. This, in combination with anxiety over the need to seek treatment and the inability to comprehend much of the hospital jargon, magnifies the individual's need to maintain a sense of identity. "Good morning, Mr. Torres; I'm Lynn Smith, the radiographer" is more than an example of good manners. It shows respect and concern and allows the patient to choose how he or she wishes to be addressed. In an effort to show friendliness, some staff may address adults as "honey" or "sweetie" instead of calling them by name. Others, who are focused on the work routine, may refer to "the gallbladder in room 2" or "that barium enema in the hall." Talking down to adults or treating them impersonally diminishes their self-esteem and raises feelings of resentment. Such feelings diminish patients' ability to understand and follow directions, prevent retention of information, and may hinder recovery.

Another way to minimize these problems is to involve patients in their own care by giving them opportunities to make choices. Avoid the false sort of choice expressed by such statements as, "Would you like to come down for your x-ray now?" When the patient is scheduled for 10 AM, little choice is involved. Valid choices require a little more thought, but the rewards in terms of patient satisfaction are well worth the effort. They do not need to be major decisions. Questions such as, "Would you like a blanket over your knees?" and "Would you prefer to sit where you can see down the hall or by the window?" reassure the patient who would like to feel capable of making decisions and having a share in his or her own care. Treating patients as individuals, allowing them to make valid choices, and using good nonverbal communication are all ways to alleviate fear.

In determining why patients fail to follow instructions, a factor frequently encountered is the assumption that the patient has understood the procedure. To make an assumption is to make a guess. For example, we could assume that since you are reading this text, you are a student in a radiologic technology training program. This may be true, or you may be an instructor, a nurse, or the proofreader for this book. Making assumptions about patients forces you to guess their physical status and abilities and also their willingness to cooperate. Can you assume that Mr. White, who may have broken his ankle, can be positioned flat on the radiographic table? No. He may have emphysema, which would interfere with his ability to breathe, or any one of many conditions that could cause difficulties in positioning.

The avoidance of assumptions becomes rather critical when ambulatory patients come in for procedures involving preparation. For example, Ms. Elwood is scheduled for cholecystography today. An inquiry such as, "Did you take those tablets before you came?" may not be a very effective way to find out what Ms. Elwood actually did. It implies that she was given the tablets, received clear instructions, and was able to comply. If you rephrase the question and ask, "What did you do to get ready for today's examination?" you may only learn that she has washed her hair and taken a shower. Reviewing the printed instructions with the patient will give you a more complete picture of how well she was able to cooperate.

When you are responsible for direct patient teaching, the approach is very similar. Involve the patient in the planning whenever possible. After the teaching period, set aside a question-and-answer session and ask the patient to explain or demonstrate the principles to you. This validation of instructions makes patients feel involved in their care, promotes their sense of autonomy, and increases compliance with the medical regimen.

Conversing with patients allows you to use your powers of observation. How alert or confused is the patient? How well does the patient hear? Is English comprehension a problem? From observation, you can often make a tentative assessment of the patient's ability to get on and off the examination table, walk unassisted to the bathroom, and so forth. In Chapter 4 we discuss patient assessment in depth, but you should learn from this chapter that good communication with patients can help you establish a spirit of trust and cooperation that will assist in patient care.

Patients who do not speak English

Language barriers are not handled very effectively in the United States. Recent federal legislation has addressed the patient's right to understand and communicate effectively in health care situations regardless of language barriers. Most large hospitals now have a facility that arranges for the services of interpreters. In areas where languages other than English are typically used, the admitting and emergency areas must post signs in the most common languages advising patients of the availability of interpreters. In many cases, certified interpreters are "on call" and come immediately when needed. When a large percentage of the population speaks a single foreign language, full-time interpreters may be part of the hospital staff. If an outpatient procedure is scheduled in advance, an interpreter may be scheduled at the same time.

The difference between a certified interpreter and a friend or family member who assumes this role may be significant. The interpreter is trained to translate only what has been said, both by the patient and to the patient, and not to explain what is implied. Family and friends may tend to add extraneous information or to edit the conversation in an effort to be cooperative or to save time. For example, a complete explanation of positioning and when to stop and start breathing may be abbreviated in translation to, "It's OK, Mama. Just hold still." Family members may hesitate to reveal information about the patient that they believe is private or embarrassing. The patient may hesitate to reveal personal information through family or friends. Family members whose command of English is limited may have good intentions but be unable to provide adequate translation of complex information. The services of a trained interpreter provide a professional bridge in difficult communication situations. Personal relationships do not interfere, and the parties to the conversation can be certain that the translations are accurate. Your duty may be to arrange for an interpreter when appropriate, even though a "family translator" may be present and this may result in a delay of routine procedures that disrupts your schedule.

When using an interpreter, look directly at the patient and speak as though the patient were able to understand you. The interpreter will translate as you speak or as soon as you have finished a sentence. Speaking to the interpreter directly tends to make the patient feel left out or talked about rather than involved in the process.

Telephone translation services, including unusual languages and obscure dialects, are available through the American Telephone and Telegraph (AT & T) long-distance service. Telephone translation is usually most efficient when a conference call format is used, but translators are patient if the telephone must be transferred from client to health care worker in the course of the conversation. If your hospital subscribes to this service or a similar one, you will receive specific instructions about its use. This method may be very effective for obtaining a medical history or informed consent when translation is otherwise not available.

One hospital emergency room near a seaport maintains a file in six languages with phrases such as, "Please hold your breath," "Point to where it hurts," and other appropriate statements. If no translator is available, it is helpful to use demonstrations or pencil sketches, validate whether the individual understands, and make extensive use of nonverbal encouragement. A friendly smile and a warm touch may be worth many words.

Impaired vision

Most of us depend greatly on our eyes to sense our surroundings and ensure our safety as we move about. Vision enables us to recognize individuals and locate items of daily living. Blind persons' ability to accomplish these same tasks without vision can seem astounding. They rely on hearing and touch to a much greater extent than sighted persons. With the aid of a cane or Seeing Eye dog, many blind persons lead very independent lives. Having learned to work outside the home, use public transportation, and maintain their own households, these patients may be insulted by attitudes that are too solicitous. On the other hand, they may welcome some special help in a strange environment. Some patients prefer to follow you by listening to your footsteps and using a cane, whereas others may wish to place a hand on your shoulder or elbow. Those who are more infirm may prefer your arm around their waist while you reassure and direct them verbally. None of these approaches applies to all blind persons. Good communication is the key to determining which form of help is acceptable and appropriate.

The person with recently failing vision and good hearing may need much verbal explanation and reassurance. Other visually impaired individuals are quite capable of proceeding confidently after a quick description of a room and the obstacles in it. You might say, "This is a square room Mrs. Daley. The x-ray table is about 5 feet in front of you, and a chair is at 7 o'clock. After you're on the table, I'll be in a booth to your left." Patients with failing vision see better in bright light. They may be able to recognize faces, but you may need to read written material to them.

Impaired hearing

In the past, many health care providers have treated deaf patients and those with some hearing loss essentially the same. In reality the problems of communication are very different. Patients with a hearing loss may display levels of impairment that vary from the need to use a high-intensity hearing aid to only a mild difficulty hearing voices in a high or low register.

Hearing loss. Certain rules are helpful in communicating with individuals with hearing loss:
1. Talk *to*, not *about*, these persons, and have their attention before starting to speak.
2. Face the person, preferably with light on your face.
3. Hearing loss is frequently in the upper register, so lower your voice when you increase the volume.
4. Speak clearly and at a moderate pace. Do not shout.
5. Avoid noisy background situations.
6. Rephrase when you are not understood.
7. Be patient.

When in doubt, ask the person for suggestions to improve communication. Avoid potential misunderstandings by using open-ended questions and requesting patients to repeat instructions.

Allow the patient who wears a hearing aid to retain it as long as possible, and give all instructions before the aid is placed in a safe location. Since visual clues become much more essential when hearing is impaired, try not to remove the patient's glasses until necessary.

Deafness. The deaf patient, unlike one with a hearing loss, presents a different set of problems. Many totally deaf individuals live in a cultural setting that has its own social structure, language, and even "inside" jokes. Certain cues help in differentiating between the patient with a hearing loss and the deaf patient, especially in an emergency. You may become aware that a seemingly alert patient is totally deaf when he or she:
1. Does not respond to noises or words spoken out of the range of vision
2. Uses lip movements without making a sound or speaks in a flat or unintelligible monotone
3. Points to the ears and mouth while shaking the head in a negative motion
4. Uses gestures or writing motions to express the need for paper and pencil

Some deaf people are adept at lip reading and are able to speak, at least to a limited degree. More often the deaf are educated in American Sign Language (ASL), which is the most common sign language and is distinctly different from English. It has a unique grammar, syntax, and rules. Learning a few basic signs may aid in establishing rapport with deaf patients. A card showing the alphabet and more useful signs in ASL should be available through your nursing service department. An interpreter is essential in any situation that requires complex instruction or an exchange of information.

When an interpreter is available, the patient should be advised that this service is provided without charge. The interpreter explains that all information is confidential and that interpretation is part of the medical service.

Interpreters for deaf clients use the same ethical guidelines as the foreign language translators discussed earlier in this chapter. Friends and relatives of a

deaf patient should *not* be used to interpret medical or treatment information. The interpreter should be used when:
1. Obtaining the patient's medical history
2. Obtaining informed consent or permission for treatment
3. Giving a diagnosis
4. The patient is conscious during treatment or surgery
5. Confronting an emergency
6. Explaining medication instructions, side effects, and dosages
7. Physicians or medical staff are giving instructions
8. The patient is being discharged

When a totally deaf patient is admitted for care, the chart should be flagged with this information. The deaf person has the right to request a specific interpreter, if available, and to have an interpreter replaced if communication is not proceeding well. Patients also have the right to choose the most preferred method of communication, which might be pencil and paper. Be sure that writing materials are available and that the patient's writing arm is free.

The medical setting can seem overwhelming to anyone, especially when the patient is a deaf child. If possible, allow the child and parents to tour the area before the examination begins. Take time to explain fully the procedures and activities to the parents so they can help the child know what to expect. If the child is distressed, you might consider allowing a parent to stay in sight or near the child, using the proper safety precautions.

Aphasia

For the patient with aphasia (the inability to speak), it is especially helpful to ask the nursing staff how they have dealt with this problem. Some patients prefer to write. Many can indicate by a nod or shake of the head whether or not they understand your directions.

Remember that the loss of the ability to see, hear, or speak is a communication impairment and not a reflection of the individual's ability to think. Patients with sensory deprivation challenge us to be more flexible and innovative in the way we offer explanation and reassurance.

Impaired mental function

Special sensitivity is needed in dealing with patients who are mentally or emotionally handicapped. Such patients may include those with congenital defects such as trisomy 21 (Down's syndrome), victims of accidents, those with illnesses affecting the brain, and those with severe emotional disorders that affect comprehension. As with children, you must assess the patient's ability to understand and follow instructions, since this ability may vary from a near infantile response to a functional capability close to normal. In general the same clear, simple, and direct instructions offered to children are appropriate. You may need to repeat instructions if the attention span is short. It is *not* appropriate to talk to these patients as if they were toddlers. Use the adult form of address, and treat them with the respect and dignity due anyone their age.

Altered states of consciousness

Another challenge to communication may arise with patients who have an altered state of consciousness. This change in the ability to respond, react, and cooperate may result from injury, illness, or medication. The impairment may range from a state of drowsiness, in which the individual can cooperate when aroused, to total unconsciousness. You must remember two points in dealing with these patients: (1) do not rely on those who are drowsy or stuporous to remember instructions, and (2) realize they are not responsible for their actions or answers. The individual who has loss of consciousness may seem to respond appropriately on regaining consciousness but may also attempt to stand or get down from the table. Any patient with decreased level of consciousness (LOC) should be kept under close observation.

An important factor frequently overlooked in hospitals is the ability of many patients to hear and remember conversations that occurred while they were apparently unconscious. Patients who are comatose because of anesthesia, trauma, or illness may be completely unable to respond but retain the ability to hear and remember what is said. A safe rule to follow is not to make any statements within hearing range of unconscious patients that you would not make if they were conscious. As a corollary to this, it is important to refer to unconscious patients by name and to reassure them about your actions. Medical literature gives many examples of patients who have regained consciousness after prolonged periods and have credited their recovery to health professionals who continued to call them by name and treat them as human beings with an identity uniquely their own.

Children and adolescents

The fear and lack of comprehension that we often see in adults are greatly magnified in children. Small children, who may have difficulty expressing themselves, respond to a friendly smile and a consistently firm, gentle, and reassuring touch. Try to find out what the child is called at home and use the familiar name. If you are calm, cheerful, and unhurried, the child is much less likely to respond negatively to the strange surroundings and machines. Allowing the small child to take a favorite blanket or toy to the radiology department may help promote a feeling of security (Fig. 2-4). Talk to small children. Even if they do not understand all you say, a cheerful voice is reassuring. Strange adults are often intimidating to children because of their stature. Try to speak to children at their own eye level. You will find that this is most effective when you approach the child to "make friends" before entering the x-ray room.

Children over the age of 4 or 5 years require somewhat different approaches to communication. They are able to share information with you and cooperate more fully, but they also fear a loss of self-control and need to make valid choices even more than do adults. "Would you like to climb up on the table by yourself or would you like me to help you?" is an example (Fig. 2-5). Although children have no choice about submitting to the examination, they should be encouraged to cooperate as much as possible. Apprehensive children are not reassured by such statements as, "This won't hurt a bit." All too frequently the only word they assimilate is "hurt," and they become even more frightened.

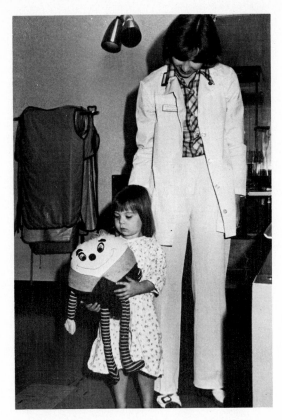

Fig. 2-4. "Humpty wants to come with me."

"Have you ever had your picture taken by x-ray?" allows you to add whatever simple explanation is necessary. "We're going to take a picture of your leg with this special big camera" is understandable to most children. Since children love to imitate adult behaviors, a demonstration is often more effective than verbal instruction. *Show* the child how to position the hand for a finger examination or how to hold a deep breath for a chest radiograph. If questions are asked, try to answer them simply. Never force information on children, since they frequently become more apprehensive if they do not understand everything that is said. It is better to treat the entire procedure in a matter-of-fact manner. Keep directions and explanations simple, direct, and honest, "We need to take five or six pictures, Johnny. We'll be as fast as we can."

How do you cope with the child who appears determined to be disruptive or refuses to follow directions? You set limits in clear terms, saying, "You must lie still," or "You may not get down." Above all, use praise for any attempt to cooperate. Every effort you make to calm a child's fear and enlist cooperation is worthwhile as long as you are making progress. Do not hesitate to ask for more experienced help in dealing with a difficult situation. If, after a patient and reasonable attempt, the child continues to resist you and the examination, you

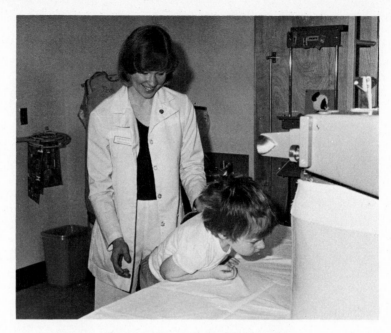

Fig. 2-5. "I can do it all by myself."

should assume that no cooperation is possible. Immobilize the patient firmly but gently, and complete the examination as quickly as you can. (See Chapter 3 for immobilization technique.)

You should remember that muscular activity is a natural response to anxiety in a small child. When the situation seems unbearable, kicking and squirming are quite normal. Crying also is normal for a frightened child. An order to stop crying only increases the anxiety, and trying to raise your voice over a child's screams is almost never effective. Sometimes, however, a whisper captures a distressed child's curiosity and attention.

Special sensitivity is also required to deal with younger adolescents' emotional needs. Although they may act quite adult under normal circumstances, they become frightened and confused and may revert to childlike behavior when ill or in stressful situations. At this age, modesty and privacy are of paramount importance. X-rays may be feared as the "all-seeing eye," ready to unveil the patient's innermost secrets.

A professional approach, coupled with warm reassurance, promotes a more positive attitude in both child and adolescent. Many poor attitudes toward health care displayed by adults may be traced to lack of sensitive care by health professionals in these adults' early years.

Older adults

Older patients may require special attention because of the physical problems that often accompany aging. The visual and hearing problems discussed previously may have direct application to many of these patients. Good lighting and checking to ensure the patient has glasses or hearing aid available helps both of you feel more comfortable. A typical attribute of aging is a tendency to proceed at one's own pace, both mentally and physically. Most older patients do not respond well to feeling pushed or hurried.

Occasionally, you will see older people who have lost varying degrees of the ability to understand why they have been placed in unfamiliar surroundings. This may be caused by Alzheimer's disease or organic brain syndrome or may occur as a direct result of medication, illness, or injury. Older patients who appear confused respond best to familiar situations. In these cases especially, use an individual's full name. During conversation, it helps to ask where the person was born, whether from a large family, and other questions about the past. Distant memory is frequently clear when a person can no longer recall what was served for breakfast. Keep instructions simple and give them one at a time. Using valid choices and treating aged patients with the respect due any adult helps them maintain their sense of identity. We emphasize that relatively few older patients have these conditions, and it is essential to evaluate each older patient's individual needs.

COMMUNICATION WITH PATIENTS' FAMILIES

When we are sick or injured, the presence of those who care about us is very reassuring and may be essential to our ability to cope. It is natural that family members accompany patients to their appointments, rush to the emergency room after an accident, and visit patients during hospital admissions. You will often have to deal with family members who want to hold the patient's hand during a radiographic examination or who eagerly await the results of a diagnostic procedure. When you are busy and the patient is your primary concern, family members may appear as obstacles to your work. Dealing sensitively with families is often necessary and helps your patient in ways that may not be apparent.

Your communication with families often involves the transfer of practical information. Those waiting for a patient want to know how long the procedure will take, and they appreciate an update from you when a delay occurs. When the wait is prolonged, your attention to the waiting family's comfort might include directions to needed services such as the restrooms, cafeteria, or telephone.

If the patient is a minor, is incompetent, or is sedated, you may need to provide instructions to a family member regarding preparations or follow-up care. Be sure you are speaking to the person who will actually assist the patient, since information can be lost when it is passed from person to person.

Questions often arise regarding the immediate presence of family members during a procedure. The family usually must stay outside the room, preferably in a waiting area or lobby that is out of hearing range. This is done not only because of radiation safety, but also because it allows the staff to proceed without interruptions from concerned family members who may not understand what is happening and may require explanations and reassurance. Procedures that involve patient discomfort or some blood loss may be very unsettling to loved ones. If families are waiting near the procedure room, you should be aware of this and avoid making statements within hearing that might alarm them or betray a professional confidence.

Occasionally a family member may need to stay with the patient in the procedure room, as with the deaf child mentioned earlier. In these situations, only one family member should be selected, and this person should receive a clear explanation before the procedure. You should answer questions at this point and clarify the family's role. A lead apron or other radiation shielding can be provided as necessary.

Sometimes dealing with families can be especially difficult. In an emotionally charged situation, we all use different means to cope with our anxiety. Some of us become dependent and wait for others to make decisions and give us instructions. Others maintain self-control by withdrawing or denying the importance of the situation. Anxiety can cause some individuals to be quite aggressive when asking personnel for information about patients who are dear to them. Families of patients in emergency situations naturally experience fear and anxiety, and these feelings may be displaced onto the closest professional person, possibly you. "Watch what you're doing." "You can't move him, he's hurt." "Are you in charge?" "Do you know what you're doing?" Such statements can elicit a negative reaction unless you recognize their hidden message. Necessary activities, such as filling out insurance forms and calling other family members, serve to bridge the waiting period. Let families know when the patient will be moved and where the patient will be going. Although you usually should refer inquiries directly to the physician in charge, an expression of concern can show empathy here. "I know how worried you must be about Barbara, Mr. Rudd; I've let the doctor know you're waiting for the results." Fear frequently engenders anger. If you can understand aggressive demands for service and attention as being an expression of fear, you can concentrate on reassuring rather than responding with anger yourself.

If families do not respond to your reasonable attempts to calm them and are preventing you from doing your work, you need help from someone who is in a better position to deal with them. Security personnel may be summoned to intervene with hostile or belligerent relatives. The social services department may send a counselor or chaplain to assist those who are grief-stricken or in a state of panic.

COMMUNICATIONS WITH CO-WORKERS

The ability to relay information to other health professionals is essential in the multidisciplinary situation existing in modern hospitals. Many problems we encounter when dealing with patients are also met when communicating with professional workers. The pressures of time and patient load may cause or compound the personality conflicts encountered in any group. Good interpersonal relationships are built on the ability to make others feel good about themselves. The nonverbal behaviors that we use with patients, such as touch and appearance, are equally effective with co-workers. Use praise and appreciation as pos-

itive reinforcements for work well done. Be a good listener, and avoid cliques
and gossip to demonstrate your respect for your co-workers as individuals. Because good communication with your co-workers is so important, we urge you
to review the principles presented earlier in this chapter and to practice them in
all your professional encounters.

In today's world a great amount of technical information is exchanged. Although much of this is conveyed using charts and forms, informal messages
may be equally important. Attention to details, such as adding your name and
the date to telephone message forms, keeps information retrieval more accurate.

Here are some guidelines for avoiding problems with telephone communications:

1. Be familiar with your telephone system, including forwarding and "hold"
   functions.
2. Identify yourself and your department when calling *or* answering a call.
3. Keep paper handy and make notes during the call to avoid losing details.
4. Use a pleasant, receptive tone of voice.
5. Validate the message before concluding the call.
6. Be sure the message is relayed to the proper person or department.

Most institutions offer video presentations to assist you in learning the correct use of the telephone in the hospital setting.

Many troublesome situations can be avoided by maintaining a pleasant working relationship that allows you to solve small problems before they grow to departmental size. Recurring problems should be handled following the chain of
command discussed in Chapter 1.

Medical information and records

Effective documentation of information about patients and their care marks the
professional who recognizes efficient record keeping as a way to meet ongoing
patient needs. Attention to clerical details may seem to be a nonprofessional
function, but dates, account numbers, chart numbers, social security numbers,
and similar data are necessary to your institution and the patients it serves. Different forms and data are used to meet various departments' needs, and your
involvement with them will vary with the agency in which you are employed,
but the principles remain the same. Any written records you initiate must be
accurate, pertinent, and *legible.*

Health care providers today use computers extensively for clerical functions
(Fig. 2-6). The storage of computer data on patients creates an individual file
for each patient. Access to these files supplies basic information about the patient, such as room number, birth date, medical record number, and next of
kin. Computer files can be used for scheduling, generating requisitions, or entering charges when procedures have been completed. However, computers are
only capable of using the information provided them. If a date is incomplete or
a name misspelled, the computer is unable to right the error and may reject the
entire entry. Most hospitals provide in-service instruction applicable to their
computer systems.

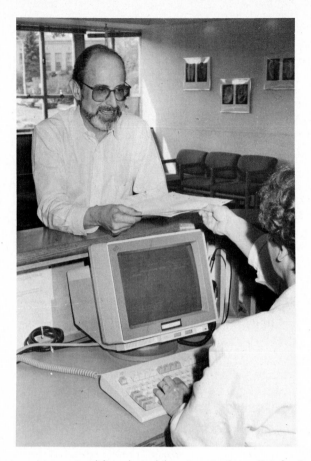

Fig. 2-6. A computer simplifies clerical functions in the radiology department.

Responsibilities for record keeping

Health care agencies are also businesses. Proper record keeping is required to ensure that patients are billed accurately, that supplies are ordered to replace those used, and that insurance companies receive verification of the care given to their clients. Failure to process information accurately and promptly may inconvenience your co-workers and pose serious problems for patients.

The chief reason for keeping accurate, pertinent medical records is to provide data about the patient's progress and current status for other health team members. Not only does this prevent the need for repetitious diagnostic examinations of the patient by various professionals, but it encourages a systematic approach to therapeutic care, allowing for longitudinal comparisons that aid in a more comprehensive approach to extended health care. Well-kept records also serve as a resource for research investigations.

Accountability is an essential term when referring to the medicolegal aspects of patient care. We cannot overemphasize the importance of correct record keeping. Above all, medical records should be objective. For example, do not chart "patient is confused" because this does not demonstrate how you came to this conclusion. "Patient appears unable to relate why he is in hospital and who or what brought him here" is a clearer statement. Objectivity is particularly important when dealing with situations that have a strong potential for legal action, such as motor vehicle accidents. "Too drunk to climb on x-ray table" is an unvalidated clinical judgment. "Appeared uncoordinated, staggered severely, and was unable to climb on x-ray table without assistance; strong odor of alcohol on breath and clothing" is an objective statement.

Poor medical records are often a major contributing factor when a defensible court case is lost. Charting should be complete, objective, consistent, legible, and accurate. The following list alerts you to some rules for avoiding mistakes frequently found when charts are audited.

1. To delete an entry, simply draw a line through it; do not erase or use correction fluid.
2. Always initial and date corrections.
3. Never leave blanks on forms. Insert "NA" or "0."
4. Never insert loose or gummed slips of paper.
5. Always include the year when dating written materials.

The chart is a legal document that can substantiate or refute charges of negligence or malpractice and can also serve as a record of behavior, which may set a precedent for the future. The course of treatment and quality of care are reflected in the chart.

The chart as a resource

Earlier in this chapter we discussed the need to validate impressions in assessing the status of patients in the radiology department. The chart is frequently your most accessible resource. Although the organization of charts may vary somewhat, certain elements are consistent. The diagnosis or "impression" is found at the conclusion of the history sheet. The patient's current status is found in the physician's progress notes and in the nurses' notes. Allergic sensitivities are usually indicated in red on the chart cover and are also stated in the history sheet. Laboratory reports, radiology reports, and results of other studies are found in a separate section, whereas the medication record may be in the nurse's notes or on a separate record near the temperature sheet. The recording of pulse, blood pressure, and temperature on a graph form allows for a longitudinal comparison.

To reduce the time involved in the charting process, as well as the volume of hospital records, charting is a somewhat streamlined form of written communication. Many frequently used words are abbreviated, and comments are made in the form of brief phrases rather than complete sentences. Some practice is needed for beginners to translate this jargon accurately. The lists of abbreviations and terms in Appendix C are helpful to students learning to use medical charts.

Problem-oriented medical recording

Problem-oriented medical recording (POMR) is a system of problem identification that started with systems analysis and is now used for medical, social, psychiatric, and demographic investigations. This system has been adapted to provide faster and more accurate medical information retrieval. To use this system, one must collect data, evaluate them and form a problem list, determine what intervention is appropriate, carry out the plan, and evaluate the results. Traditional charts include a running commentary on the patient's total condition. Since most patients have several problems, retrieval of information on a specific point is rather cumbersome. Suppose Mr. Clark has been admitted with hypertension but also has dermatitis and mild diarrhea. In traditional charts, you would need to comb through the nurses' notes and/or progress record and/or graph sheet to see if diarrhea is an immediate problem that will complicate today's radiographic examination. Using POMR, you may look at the list of problems in the front of the chart, find the number assigned to the problem that concerns you, and then look for that number in the joint progress notes kept by all medical staff providing care (Fig. 2-7).

When you look for information on a specific problem, you will find the letters S, O, A, and P in the margin with a narrative next to each letter. These initials stand for the words subjective, objective, assessment, and plan. *Subjective* observations are symptoms and personal reactions related by the patient. *Objective* observations are the signs and measurements that can be substantiated by the observer, such as weight, temperature, laboratory results, and emesis. *Assessment* is the definition of the problem, such as "obese—50 pounds overweight" or "diarrhea secondary to medication reaction." *Plan* is what the health provider intends to do to deal with the problem.

In essence, this charting system allows identification of each of the patient's

		PROBLEM LIST		
Date identified	Date of onset	Problem number	Problem title	Date inactive/ resolved
9-12-92	8-90	1	hypertension	
9-12-92	−'86	2	Obesity	12-21-92
1/4/93	1/2/93	3	dehydration − persistent emesis	
1/5/93	1/5/93	4	R.L.2 pain	

Fig. 2-7. A, Problem list used with problem-oriented medical recording (POMR).

REDLAND VALLEY HOSPITAL PROGRESS NOTES			Joeckle, Albert 763-91-93 8-14-30 Dr. M.Erbele

Date	Time	Problem #	Progress Note
1/5/93 Cont.	900	3	S. Continues to complain of nausea and abdominal discomfort which he blames on new medication O. T-99⁶ P86 apical R-18 A/P increasing Gastro intestinal upset. Dr. Erbele notified
	1130	3	S. unable to tolerate clear liquid diet O. Emesis 60cc clear bile Tinged fluid P. Compazine suppository Ī given per VO Dr. Erbele
	1240		O. sleeping E Wryn RN
1/5/93	1540	4	S. Complains of Rt Ʒ pain states he's unable to stand straight due to pain O T-101⁶ P 90 R 20 Rebound tenderness RLƷ A ʃ oss. appendicitis P. notify her. Erbele Warrick Lawera NP

S- Subjective data (symptoms)
O-Objective data (measurable signs)
A-Assessments (conclusions)

P- Plan—immediate or future
I- Intervention—action
E- Evaluation—effectiveness of intervention

Fig. 2-7—cont'd. B, Example of joint progress notes using POMR.

problems. It permits differentiation between long-term and short-term problems, enabling you to focus on the immediate situation without ignoring long-term goals. (Reducing obesity, increasing exercise tolerance, or giving up smoking would be examples of long-term goals for the hypertensive patient.) POMR also permits ease of retrieval for specific information, such as cost analysis, quality control, and research, and remains the legal record of the course and quality of care.

Medical recording by radiographers

Requisitions and reports are forms of particular importance to radiographers. An x-ray requisition serves as the formal order for a diagnostic procedure. It includes patient data, a brief medical history, and specific instructions. In some situations it may be part of a multicopy form that eventually may include the radiologist's report. Both the requisition and the report are medicolegal records and may be filed with the films or separately. The original copies of inpatient reports become part of the patient's chart. Copies of reports are also supplied directly to physicians.

Although radiographers are not responsible for initiating these records, they rely on requisitions for information about each examination they perform. They may also refer to previous reports for information about the patient's problem or the radiologist's recommendations for further studies.

Medical recording by radiographers varies greatly from one institution to another, and you must become familiar with your facility's requirements. Documenting certain information about patients is an essential part of the medicolegal record. This includes administration of contrast media or medications, changes in patient status, and reactions to contrast or medications, as well as any treatment in the radiology department. Examples of such treatment include oxygen given to a patient who becomes short of breath or hot packs applied to an intravenous (IV) site when an IV line has extravasated.

Inpatient charts usually accompany patients to the radiology department. The chart is usually where you record changes in status, medications, and treatments. In your hospital the information to be recorded might be placed in chart pages titled "Nurses' Notes," "Progress Notes," or "Medication Records." In some departments completion of the procedure is routinely charted by the radiographer in the nurses' notes. The information you chart should include the date, the time (using the 24-hour clock; e.g., 2:15 PM is charted as 1415), a specific statement of what occurred, and your signature. When charting observations or treatments on behalf of the radiologist, include the radiologist's name followed by a slash mark and your signature. Although nurses often use only initials to identify their entries, they are part of a small group repeatedly using the chart, and their initials with their full name are recorded elsewhere in the chart for legal verification. When radiographers chart, they should use a full signature and a designation of the department or position so that identification is clear.

An increasing proportion of the patients seen in imaging departments are outpatients who do not have a chart per se, but accurate medical records are important for these patients as well. Your observations must be recorded on the proper form, which will be filed with either the report or the films. Initials may be adequate identification for routine notes on records generated in your own department. Complete signatures, however, are needed for witnessing documents such as informed consents, consents to treatment, and incident reports.

Radiographs as records

Radiographs are a part of the medicolegal record and are considered the property of the institution in which they are made. Patients often assume that because they have paid for the examination, the films belong to them. Tact is required when explaining that the charges cover the expense of the procedure and that every effort will be made to ensure the films are available when needed to assist in the patient's care.

State laws vary with respect to the length of time radiographs must legally be kept on file. Usually the retention period is 5 to 7 years, with the additional requirement that films on minors be kept 5 to 7 years after the patient reaches majority, or legal age (18 to 21 years, depending on the state).

Since charts can easily be photocopied, the original is never allowed to leave the health facility. Radiographs are more difficult to duplicate, however, and the quality is never equal to that of the original. For this reason it is often helpful for original films to be made available for comparison or consultation outside the institution of origin. This is not necessarily true with computer-assisted imaging modalities, in which laser cameras now permit more than one original copy of each film to be made. Since rules governing confidentiality also apply to radiographs, the patient must sign a release form when films are needed by another provider. A written record of the date and the borrower's name and address meets the legal obligation to keep the films on file. Usually, follow-up procedures exist to ensure return of films that have been loaned, but films are sometimes checked out for indefinite periods, as when a patient with a chronic condition moves to another state.

It is usually recommended that films be sent directly to a consulting physician rather than allowing the patient to transport them. Sometimes, however, it is more convenient for the patient to carry the films. In this case a physician should view the films with the patient and answer any questions in advance, since the patient's curiosity may result in an attempt to interpret the films. This may lead to unnecessary confusion and anxiety. For example, patients have been known to assume that a heart shadow is a lung tumor or that a gas bubble indicates a serious disease.

CONCLUSION

The progress of humankind has depended on our ability to communicate with one another. In the hospital setting, many factors cause patients anxiety and fear. When we take time to empathize, we find greater personal satisfaction in our work and improve the quality of care. The same principles of communication increase the effectiveness of our relationships with co-workers.

Charts serve as a valuable resource to the radiographer who needs to validate information on the patient's current status and record appropriate observations and procedures done in the radiology department. The ability to communicate well with patients and other health professionals is the mark of an effective professional.

Study questions

1. Draw a line representing the health-illness continuum and place the following patients appropriately on your graph.
   a. A young mother having a prenatal ultrasound study
   b. A 50-year-old male with terminal cancer
   c. A baby with pneumonia
   d. A 30-year-old obese female
   e. A 76-year-old male with a fractured ankle
2. Describe how nonverbal communication can be used with children in the radiography suite. How would you validate the effectiveness of such communication?
3. Describe five situations in which the ability to obtain information rapidly from the chart might be of critical importance.
4. Review a sample chart and identify the subjective, objective, assessment, and plan components. If these items are not in a SOAP format, make a sample progress note using this system.

3

Safety, Transfer, and Positioning

Objectives

At the conclusion of this chapter, the student will be able to:

1. List three common infractions of fire safety rules in hospitals.
2. List four important electrical safety precautions.
3. List in sequence the steps to be taken if you discover a fire in or near the radiology department.
4. Discuss hazards caused by obstructions and spills.
5. List two steps to be taken to ensure accuracy of patient identification.
6. Demonstrate safe techniques for patient moving and transferring, using the principles of good body mechanics:
   a. Assist patient to sit from a recumbent position.
   b. Assist patient into and out of wheelchair.
   c. Perform two-person transfer of patient from bed to stretcher and stretcher to bed.
7. List four complications that may arise from improper patient positioning.
8. Demonstrate the use of pillows and positioning blocks to ensure the patient is comfortable on the x-ray table.
9. List three situations when the patient's head should be elevated.
10. Demonstrate proper use of safety straps, side rails, restraints, and compression bands.

Vocabulary list

1. base of support
2. center of gravity
3. debilitation
4. decubitus ulcers
5. dyspnea
6. electrical ground
7. ischial tuberosity
8. kyphotic
9. line of gravity
10. lordotic
11. orthopnea
12. orthostatic hypotension
13. premedication
14. radiolucent
15. sedation
16. spontaneous combustion

FIRE AND OTHER HAZARDS

Fire prevention

Nothing strikes terror in a hospital situation more than the word "fire." Our first discussion of safety practices is directed toward fire prevention, since it is obviously preferable to practice fire prevention than to cope with a fire. An awareness of potential hazards is the first step toward prevention.

Three components must be present for a fire to burn: a flammable substance (fuel), oxygen, and heat (Fig. 3-1). Fire can be avoided by ensuring that these three elements never occur in the same place at the same time. Conversely, a fire can be stopped if one of the elements can be removed from the situation. We use this principle when we fight a fire by adding water (lowering the temperature) or by smothering (removing oxygen), as when we wrap a blanket around a person whose clothing has ignited.

Most hospital fires are traceable to one of four causes:

1. Spontaneous combustion
2. Open flames
3. Smokers
4. Electricity

Spontaneous combustion occurs when a chemical reaction in or near a flammable material causes sufficient heat to generate a fire. This is a relatively infrequent cause of hospital fires, since hospital safety standards control the types of chemicals and cleaning products in general use. Since the advent of recycling, however, this has become a greater potential risk. At present it costs approximately $2500 to dispose of one barrel of chemical waste in an approved manner. Laboratories and maintenance departments now retain chemical, plastic, and glass materials for recycling in areas that may not have been designed for this purpose. Spontaneous combustion may also occur during renovations, when paint products and cleaning rags may be stored temporarily in a closed environment or too near a heat source. Oily or paint-soaked waste should be placed in tightly covered containers outside the facility. These are usually located near the maintenance department.

Open flames that burn out of control are a common source of fires in homes, but relatively few hospital fires begin in this way. Those that do usually occur in kitchens or laboratories where open burners are used. Precautions include

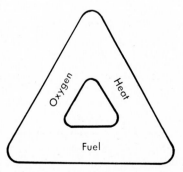

Fig. 3-1.   Chemistry of fire.

keeping flammable substances a safe distance from the flame, using strict standards of cleanliness in the kitchen, and never leaving open flames untended.

As health care providers, hospitals are attempting to promote positive health habits by prohibiting smoking. Therefore, most hospitals are designated as nonsmoking facilities, which has reduced the incidence of this type of fire. Danger still exists from covert smoking, however, because hospitals are no longer equipped to accommodate smoking. Since hospitalization tends to produce anxiety, smokers tend to cope by smoking. They must be directed to the designated smoking area, which may be outside.

Electrical failures are potential sources of fire hazard and are of special concern in radiology departments where there is much electrical equipment. For this reason, we emphasize avoiding electrical hazards and preventing electrical fires. The same principles apply in any area where electrical equipment is used, especially in the emergency room and the intensive care unit.

The following rules can be applied to reduce the likelihood of electrical fire:

1. All electrical equipment and appliances used in the hospital should be inspected and approved for hospital use by a qualified testing agency, such as the Underwriters' Laboratories (UL).

2. Follow manufacturer's instructions in using and caring for electrical equipment. Pay particular attention to whether or not a given item is washable or immersible. Improper cleansing may create a hazard.

3. All electrical equipment used in contact with patients and in areas where there is water, such as the darkroom, should be equipped with grounded (three-pronged) plugs. Equipment with three-pronged plugs must always be used with properly grounded outlets. Never use plug adapters to avoid grounding an appliance.

4. Electrical equipment must be inspected regularly. Arrange for prompt repair of any equipment that shows evidence of damage, frayed insulation, or loose plugs. Immediately discontinue use of any equipment that causes sparks or an unusual smell.

5. When fuses require replacement, always use a fuse of the proper resistance. Do not attempt to replace fuses if you are unsure about what you are doing. If fuses "blow" or circuit breakers trip repeatedly, have an electrician check all equipment on the circuit to determine and remedy the cause of the overload. This may be a sign of faulty wiring or inadequate electrical supply.

6. Always disconnect the power supply before exposing the electrical circuitry in any piece of equipment. Unplug portable units or shut off the main power switch on permanent installations.

7. Never attempt to make electrical repairs unless you have been specially trained to do so.

8. If you must use an extension cord, use the shortest cord that will do the job. Be certain that all extension cords are labeled to show their amperage capacity and are approved for hospital use. Specifications must match or exceed the capacity of the original cord attached to the equipment. Do not bring cords from home for any purpose.

9. In case of an electrical fire, use a carbon dioxide foam or Halon fire extin-

guisher. Water and some chemical extinguishers increase the hazard of electrical shock.

A short circuit in an x-ray control panel may result in fire. This is usually preceded by smoldering wire insulation, which causes smoke and an unpleasant odor, and is usually readily detectable before an actual fire. If a short circuit occurs, turn off the electricity at the main power source, call for qualified assistance, and stand by with the proper fire extinguisher. All radiographers should be aware of the locations of these extinguishers and instructed in their use.

During your education as a radiographer, you will learn to use a wide variety of complex electrical equipment. Do not let familiarity with electrical items lull you into a false sense of security.

Oxygen by itself does not burn, but it does support combustion. Since the presence of oxygen greatly increases the fire hazard, it is important to exercise extreme care when it is in use. There should be no smoking, no open flames, and no ungrounded appliances. Be familiar with the location and operation of oxygen shut-off valves in your area (Fig. 3-2).

Be prepared.   Hospitals are required to observe certain fire safety precautions to maintain their accreditation. In most hospitals the head of the maintenance

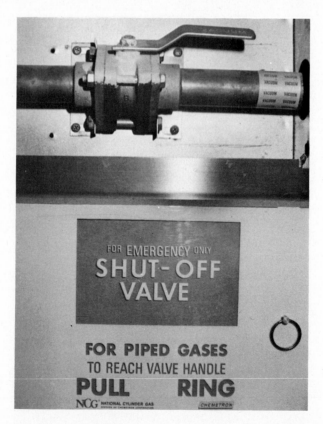

Fig. 3-2. Oxygen shut-off valve, an important location to remember.

department or the chief engineer is responsible for initiating fire safety programs. These include clearly defined plans for staff action in the event of a fire, fire drills every calendar quarter, and frequent in-service classes on procedures and firefighting equipment. The radiographer must be familiar with the fire plan for the hospital, especially for the radiology department. Be sure you know the evacuation route from your area and at least one alternate route. In addition, have at least a general knowledge of your facility's floor plan. Be certain of the location of fire alarms, fire extinguishers, and fire doors.

Fire drills must be taken seriously. In the event of a fire, a coded communication is usually used to notify the staff without alarming the patients. This may be a code number announced over the paging system: "Attention all staff, there is a code 100 on Three East." Some hospitals use a special message, such as, "Dr. Redfern, report to Third Floor East." This same code is frequently used for fire drills. Take full advantage of fire drills and in-service classes to gain confidence in evacuation procedures and the use of fire extinguishers. We hope that you will never be involved in an actual fire, but if you are well prepared, your self-confidence will allow you to function effectively and will reassure those around you.

Professional fire marshalls have stated that the most frequent infractions of fire safety rules include blocking fire doors to prevent them from closing, storing equipment in corridors, improperly storing flammable items, and using extension cords not approved for hospital use.

Fire doors are designed and constructed to restrict the spread of a fire to a small area. For this reason, fire doors should never be blocked open. They should remain closed unless they are of the type designed to close automatically when the fire alarm is activated.

Since radiographers often use mobile stretchers, wheelchairs, carts, and x-ray machines, care must be taken to avoid obstructing passages and doorways. Equipment too close to a corner may be an unseen obstruction to someone hurrying from an intersecting hallway or carrying a bulky object. Corridors should not be used to store equipment, but if necessity demands that some items be placed there temporarily, keep them all on the same side and make sure that room is available to pass easily. Ask yourself the question, "If we had to evacuate the area, would this piece of equipment be a problem in this location?"

In case of fire.   If you discover a fire, your primary responsibility is to *evacuate persons in the immediate area* to a safe location beyond at least two intervening fire doors. Second, *report the fire and location,* using the prescribed code procedure. Occasionally a wastebasket blaze may be extinguished with a nearby pitcher of water or smothered with a pillow, but do not waste precious minutes in futile attempts. Report the fire as soon as the immediate area is evacuated. Hospital personnel trained in firefighting will assess the situation and direct an appropriate course of action.

The following steps also apply if the fire is in another part of the building: close all doors, shut off all electrical equipment, shut off main oxygen valves, and prepare patients for further evacuation while awaiting instruction. If the fire is in or near the radiology department, a staff member will direct patients

---

In Case of Fire

Remain calm!

1. Evacuate persons from the immediate area.
2. Report the fire and *precise* location.
3. Close all doors.
4. Shut off main oxygen valves.
5. Shut off all electrical equipment.
6. Prepare patients for further evacuation.
7. Stand by for further instruction from authorized personnel.

---

to a safe area. During evacuation, it is especially important to remain calm, use a low voice, and try to avoid using the word "fire." Instead, you might say, "Mrs. Jensen, there is a little smoke in one of the rooms, and we are going to move you outside until we can see how serious it is." The box above lists the steps to follow in case of fire.

Again, no substitute exists for knowing the location of the fire extinguishers, fire alarms (Fig. 3-3), and fire doors. Although this is usually included as part of your hospital orientation, familiarity with this information is your personal responsibility. Thorough knowledge of the prescribed procedure for reporting a fire is also essential.

Fire extinguishers.   Fires are classified according to the type of fuel involved. Class A fires involve solid combustibles such as paper or wood; class B fires,

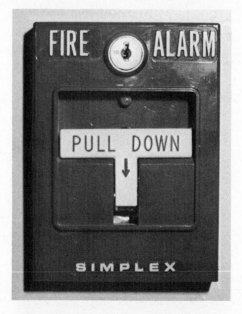

Fig. 3-3. Know this location by heart.

flammable liquids or gases; and class C fires, electrical equipment or wiring. Fire extinguishers are marked to indicate the class or classes of fire for which they are appropriately used. A multipurpose, dry chemical extinguisher is suitable for all three classes of fires and is the type most often found in hospitals and other public buildings.

Fig. 3-4 shows a close-up view of a typical fire extinguisher mechanism. To use the fire extinguisher correctly, remember the acronym PASS:

Pull the pin.
Aim the nozzle.
Squeeze the handle.
Sweep. Use a sweeping motion from side to side (Fig. 3-5).

Fire extinguishers have considerable force and are effective at a safe distance from the fire. Stand back so as not to endanger yourself.

Fire extinguishers must be inspected regularly and recharged periodically. A tag attached to the unit should indicate the dates of the last inspection and the last recharge. The last inspection should be no longer than 1 year ago. When an extinguisher has been used, it must be returned to the maintenance department to be recharged and replaced immediately with a fresh unit.

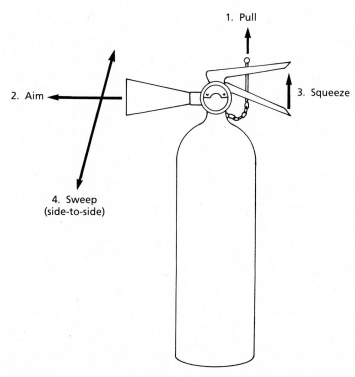

Fig. 3-4. Fire extinguisher mechanism. *1*, Pull; *2*, aim; *3*, squeeze; *4*, sweep.

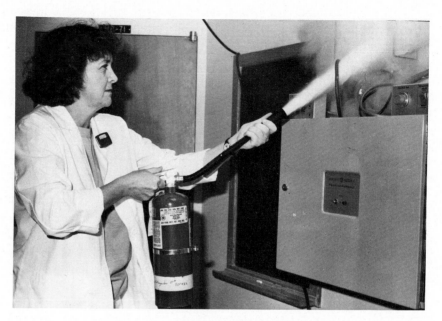

Fig. 3-5.   Use fire extinguisher in a sweeping motion from side to side.

Other common hazards

Electric shock may pose a serious hazard to both patients and personnel if safety precautions are not observed. This is especially true with x-ray equipment, which often carries an electrical potential in excess of 100,000 volts. The hazard of lesser circuits should not be underestimated, however, since shocks from standard 110-volt outlets may prove fatal under certain circumstances. The rules for reducing the likelihood of electrical fires are listed on p. 55. Adherence to these rules greatly reduces the possibility of electric shock as well. In addition, use extreme caution when using electricity around water. Never stand on a wet floor or use wet hands to perform tasks involving the use of electricity.

Take care that electrical cords are not strung across doorways or other traffic patterns. Try to position equipment as close as possible to a suitable outlet. If a cord must cross a traffic path temporarily, secure it to the floor with tape to minimize the possibility of someone tripping over it. If hazardous, makeshift electrical connections are a common problem, use the chain of command to suggest a safe, permanent remedy.

Spills deserve the special attention of the safety-conscious radiographer. Depending on the nature of the substance, spills may pose a chemical hazard in addition to the risk of injury from falls. Chemicals may be as simple as household cleaning agents or as complex as radioactive testing materials. Household bleach or concentrated darkroom chemicals may cause eye damage or skin burns. Appropriate cleaning measures are needed to avoid potentially serious problems.

Your hospital has written policies and procedures to follow in determining appropriate action in event of a chemical spill. The following steps help to ensure safety. When a spill occurs:

1. Limit access to the area.
2. Evaluate the risks involved.
3. Determine whether you have both the equipment and the expertise to clean up the spill safely.
4. If you can proceed safely, clean up the spill immediately.
5. If you lack the necessary skill or equipment, call your supervisor or the appropriate department.

BODY MECHANICS

The principles of proper body alignment, movement, and balance are referred to as body mechanics. The application of these principles minimizes the energy required to sit, stand, and walk. Your effective strength is increased when you use these principles to perform tasks that require stooping, lifting, pushing, pulling, and carrying.

Applied body mechanics also prevents muscle and back strain. Such strains are a common problem among hospital workers, causing much discomfort and reduced efficiency. Severe strains may require hospitalization and long-term therapy, with considerable pain, inconvenience, and expense. When you injure yourself on the job, you place a greater burden on the other team members. If you injure yourself while lifting a patient, you may injure the patient as well. Since an ounce of prevention is still worth a pound of cure, save your back by using your head.

Three concepts are essential to understanding the principles of body mechanics (Fig. 3-6).

The first concept is the *base of support,* which is the portion of the body in contact with the floor or other horizontal surface. It may be represented by a line drawn between the points of contact, such as between the feet when the body is erect. A broad base of support provides stability for body position and movement.

The second concept is the *center of gravity,* or center of body weight, which is the point around which body weight is balanced. It is usually located in the midportion of the pelvis or lower abdomen, but the location may vary somewhat depending on body build. Since any object you hold adds to the weight on the base of support, a load's size and position affect the location of the center of gravity. The body is most stable when the center of gravity is nearest the center of the base of support.

The third concept is the *line of gravity,* an imaginary vertical line passing through the center of gravity. The body is most stable when the line of gravity bisects the base of support.

Using these concepts, the principles of body mechanics can be stated in four simple rules. Memorizing them is easy. Smooth performance requires practice.

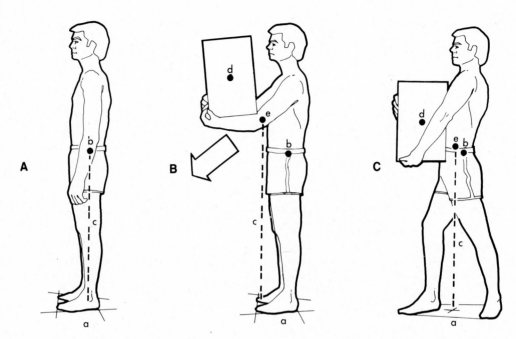

Fig. 3-6. Body mechanics. *a,* Base of support; *b,* center of gravity; *c,* line of gravity; *d,* Center of gravity of the load; *e,* combined center of gravity. **A,** With good posture, line of gravity bisects base of support. **B,** When load is held away from the body, line of gravity does *not* bisect base of support. **C,** A wide stance with load held close to the body allows combined line of gravity to bisect base of support.

⇒ Rules of body mechanics

1. Provide a wide and stable base of support. This can be easily accomplished by standing with the feet apart and one foot slightly advanced.
2. Keep your load well balanced and close to your body when lifting or carrying (Fig. 3-7). Less energy is needed to maintain your balance when the load is close to your center of gravity. Use a cart to transport any load that is reasonably heavy or must be transported any distance.
3. Keep your back straight, and avoid twisting your trunk when lifting and carrying. Plan ahead by working at a comfortable height whenever possible. Bend your knees when reaching near the floor (Fig. 3-8).
4. Use your leg and abdominal muscles when moving or lifting heavy objects. It is better to roll or push a heavy object than to use your back to pull or lift it. Remember that your thigh muscles are among the strongest in your body. By combining this strength with that of your arms and abdomen, you can avoid strain on the shorter, more vulnerable back muscles.

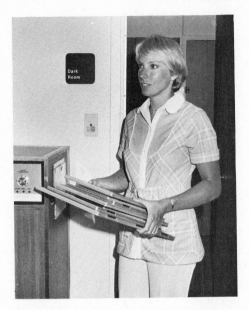

Fig. 3-7. Keep load close to your body.

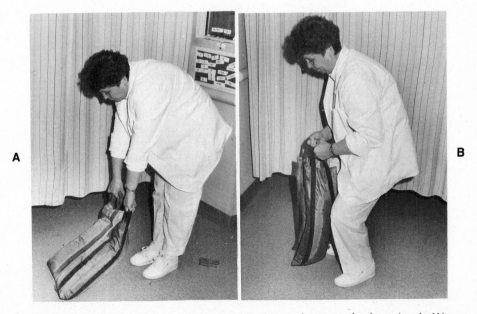

Fig. 3-8. Good body mechanics help avoid fatigue and prevent back strain. **A,** Wrong. Bend knees. **B,** Right. Keep back straight.   *Continued.*

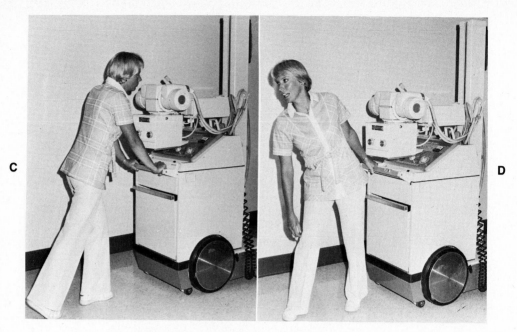

Fig. 3-8—cont'd. C, Push. **D,** Do not pull.

PATIENT TRANSFER
Preparation for transfer

The first principle of safely moving a patient is to be certain that you have the right patient. Check all identification bracelets against the requisitions, and ask patients to tell you their names as a double check.

A brief visit with patients assists in assessing how well they can help with their own transfer. This allows you to plan for additional hands, if needed, to ensure a safe move. Decide on the safest, easiest method of moving your patient, obtain the necessary equipment, and check to be certain it is functional and safe. The person transporting the patient is responsible for ensuring that the buckles on safety straps are secure, that side rails lock in the "up" position, and that brakes work properly. Move any furniture or obstacles that may be in the way.

Next, tell the patient what you plan to do and explain his or her role in the transfer. Since patients can often anticipate painful errors, the radiographer should listen carefully, allowing the patient to participate in the plan.

Wheelchair transfers

The process of transferring a patient from the bed to a wheelchair may seem elementary, but it is a common cause of falls and accidents. The correct technique makes this procedure safer and easier (Fig. 3-9). Start by lowering the bed to the level of the wheelchair seat and elevating the head of the bed. Position the wheelchair parallel to the bed with wheels locked and footrests out of the way. Place one arm under the patient's shoulders, one under the knees,

Fig. 3-9. Wheelchair transfer.

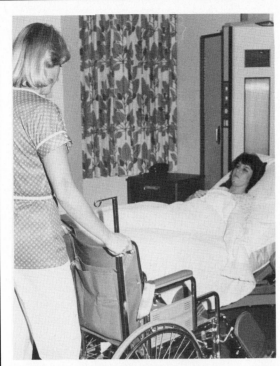

Position wheelchair parallel to patient's bed with wheels locked and footrests out of the way.

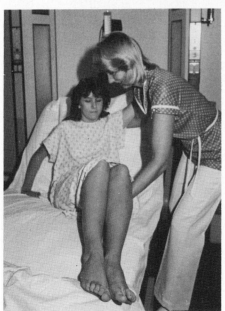

Lower bed and side rails; lift patient to a sitting position.

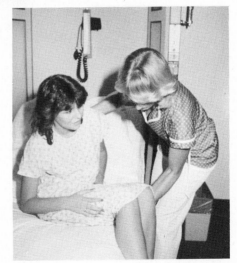

Pivot while lifting, allowing patient's legs to clear edge of bed.

Continued.

Fig. 3-9.

Wheelchair transfer—cont'd.

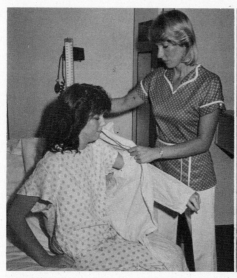

Allow patient to rest briefly before standing.

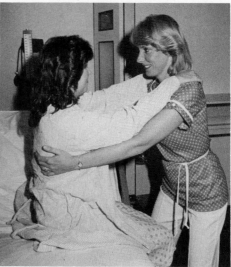

Using face-to face assist, help raise weak patient to standing position.

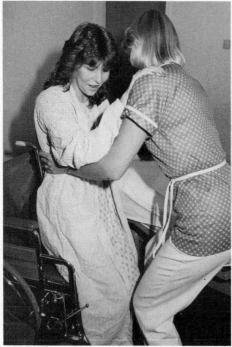

Provide support as patient eases into wheelchair.

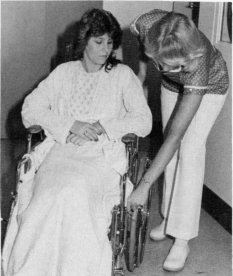

Adjust leg and footrests; cover patient's lap and legs.

and in a single, smooth motion, raise the patient to a sitting position. The patient is now sitting on the edge of the bed with the feet dangling over the side.

Take a moment at this point to assist the patient to put on slippers and robe. Many patients have *orthostatic hypotension* after long periods of rest and may feel lightheaded or faint when rising suddenly. This pause gives them an opportu-portunity to regain their sense of balance.

At this point, most competent patients are able to stand and move to the wheelchair with little assistance, although a steadying hand at the patient's elbow is a good practice. The weak patient needs additional help.

If assistance is required, stand facing the patient. Reaching around the patient, place your hands firmly over the scapulae. The patient's hands may rest on your shoulders. On your signal, lift upward, and the patient rises to a standing position. Now, pivot a quarter turn so that the edge of the wheelchair is touching the back of the patient's knees. Ease the patient into a sitting position in the chair. Position the footrests and leg rests and cover the patient's lap and knees with a sheet or bath blanket. This provides both warmth and comfort while protecting the patient's modesty.

To move the patient from wheelchair to x-ray table, place the wheelchair parallel to the table (Fig. 3-10). Lock the brakes, move footrests out of the way, and position a step stool nearby. Using the face-to-face assist explained previously, help the patient to stand. The patient now places one hand on the stool handle, puts one arm on your shoulder, and steps up onto the stool, pivoting with the back to the table. Again, ease the patient to a sitting position. Now, place one arm around the patient's shoulders and one under the knees. With a single, smooth motion, place the patient's legs on the table while lowering the head and shoulders into the supine position.

Patients who cannot stand and those who have not stood or walked since an accident, surgery, or heart attack should *not* be transported by wheelchair. These patients must not be allowed to stand or walk in the radiology department, even if they believe they are capable of doing so.

Stretcher transfers

A stretcher should be used to transport any patient who is unable to stand safely. This is also the method of choice for patients who cannot sit comfortably for an extended period. Remember, the patient may have to wait in the radiology department before or after the examination. Weak patients who cannot stand are sometimes under physicians' orders to sit in a chair as part of their daily routine. A visit to the radiology department should not be seized as an opportunity to meet this requirement. Such patients can be moved from chair to bed much more easily than from chair to x-ray table, since the table's height cannot be adjusted. If you have any doubt about the patient's ability to transfer from the chair to the table, be safe and start with a stretcher.

The following technique may be used to transfer patients to the stretcher from either the bed or the radiographic table. If the patient is able to assist and is not too heavy, you may be able to accomplish the stretcher transfer by yourself. Obtain the help of one or more other persons if the patient is obese or

Fig. 3-10.

Assisting patient onto radiographic table.

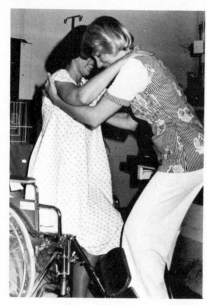

Assist patient to stand.

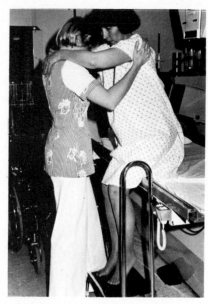

Help patient to sit on table.

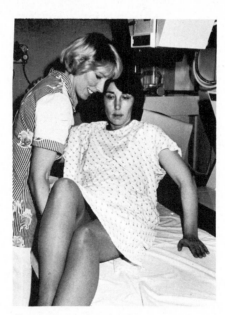

Support patient's shoulders while raising legs onto table; ease to supine position.

very weak. Provide for the patient's privacy by closing the door to the hallway or drawing the curtains between the beds. Start with the patient near the edge of the bed in the supine position, with knees flexed and feet flat. Adjust the bed to the height of the stretcher. Position the stretcher parallel to the bed and lock the wheels. Check to be certain that oxygen lines, intravenous (IV) tubing, and urinary catheters are free and will not be pulled during the transfer.

If you are working alone, lean across the stretcher, placing one arm under the patient's shoulders and the other arm under the pelvis. On your instructions, the patient pushes with feet and elbows as you lift and pull the patient toward the stretcher. Do not attempt to make the transfer in a single motion. The maneuver may be repeated several times until the transfer is complete. If you are working with an assistant, one person supports the head, neck, and shoulders while the second person lifts at the pelvis and knees (Fig. 3-11). Both use the lift-pull motion, with the patient's assistance, until the patient is safely positioned on the stretcher. Then cover the patient and secure the safety straps or side rails.

To reverse this transfer, position the stretcher parallel to the bed, lock the wheels, and release the safety straps or side rails. Since beds are wider than stretchers, it is usually better to work from the stretcher side. Position and support the patient as before. This time, on signal, the patient pushes toward the bed while you assist with a lift-push motion. Repeat as required until the transfer is complete. This same method applies to transfers from the stretcher to the x-ray table.

Various techniques are used for stretcher transfers, depending on the patient's weight and ability to assist. With problem transfers, it is best to obtain experienced help. Other methods of transfer involve the use of draw sheets and slide boards. These are often useful when the patient is unable to assist with the transfer. Practice these transfers in class before attempting to use them with patients.

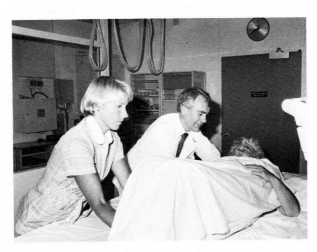

Fig. 3-11. Stretcher transfer. Allow patient to help as much as possible.

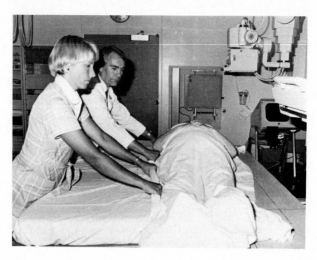

Fig. 3-12. Ready for stretcher transfer with draw sheet pull.

Patients who need frequent help with moving are often placed on a "draw" or "pull" sheet. This is a single sheet folded in half that is placed under the patient and over the middle third of the bed. When moving the patient, the edges of the draw sheet are loosened from the bed and rolled up close to the patient's body (Fig. 3-12). The rolled edge provides a handhold for lifting and pulling the patient. This method requires two or more persons. Care must be taken that the patient's head and feet move safely with the trunk of the body.

The slide board transfer is a variation of this method. It employs a strong sheet of smooth plastic, large enough to support the patient's body, with handholds cut into the board's edges. The patient is rolled to one side, and the board is slipped below the draw sheet and about halfway under the patient's body (Fig. 3-13). The remaining width of the board covers the space between the

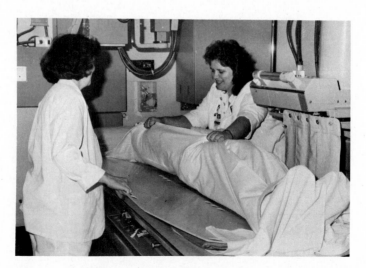

Fig. 3-13. Slide board eases stretcher transfer.

stretcher and the bed. With the patient's arms folded safely across the chest, two persons grip the draw sheet and slide the patient safely and smoothly across the board. Do *not* use flexible slide boards for spinal immobilization.

⟱ **Rules for safe patient transfer**

1. Plan what you are going to do and prepare your work area. Obtain equipment and check it for safety and function.
2. Enlist the patient's help and cooperation. Remember to tell the patient what you are doing as you proceed.
3. Obtain additional help when necessary. Check to make certain your assistants understand their role in the transfer plan.
4. Hold the patient, not the equipment.

POSITIONING FOR SAFETY AND COMFORT

It is easier to communicate with other members of the health team and to follow physicians' orders if you are familiar with the names of some of the more common body positions (Fig. 3-14).

Support and padding

When lying on a hard surface, such as an x-ray table, patients are more comfortable with radiolucent sponges or cushions strategically placed for support. If a cushion or pillow under the head will not be a hindrance to the examination, it can enable the patient to see what is occurring and thus help relieve apprehension. Elevation of the patient's head also relieves neck strain, allows easier breathing, and helps avoid the uncomfortable feeling that the head is lower than the feet. The addition of a bolster under the knees of a supine patient relieves lumbosacral stress by straightening the lordotic lumbar curve. This is especially comforting to arthritic and kyphotic patients and elderly persons.

The measures used to promote comfort are frequently the same interventions designed to prevent complications. When the body is supine, the weight of the abdominal contents pushes the diaphragm up into the thoracic cavity, making it more difficult to take a deep breath. This is no problem for most of us, but patients with *dyspnea* or *orthopnea* are unable to lie supine. A patient who becomes short of breath when supine must be assisted to sit up immediately. Patients who are nauseated also need to have their heads elevated. This position helps control nausea and prevents aspiration of emesis if the patient vomits. Patients with abdominal pain must have the head elevated and a bolster under the knees to relieve strain on the abdomen.

Padding placed under body prominences, such as the sacrum, heels, or ischial tuberosities, is important for several reasons (Fig. 3-15). One reason is that if patients are reasonably comfortable, they will be better able to maintain the positions needed for an effective examination, even on a hard surface. Another reason is that many older or debilitated patients develop ulcerated areas over prominences when pressure is exerted for any length of time. These lesions are referred to as *decubitus ulcers* or bedsores.

The cause of these problems is simple to understand and important to remember. Pressure on a limited area of tissue inhibits circulation, depriving the

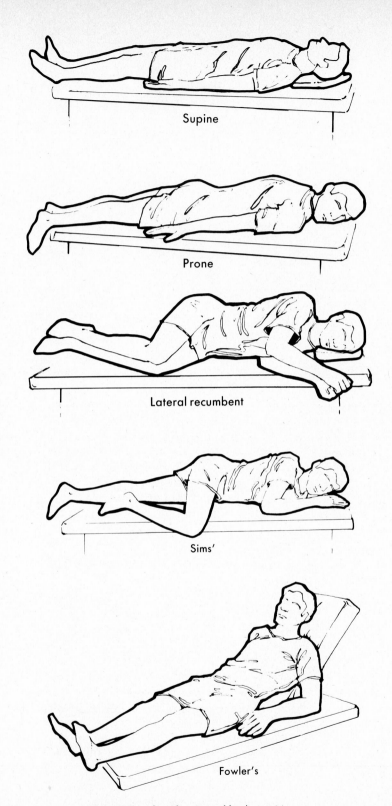

Fig. 3-14. Identification of body positions.

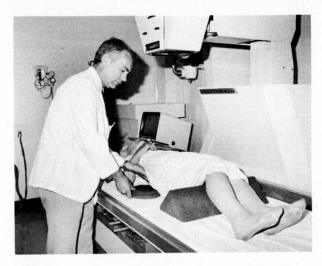

Fig. 3-15. Padding provides comfort and safety when positioning older patients.

cells of oxygen and nutrition. The cells in the middle of the area are affected first. If the pressure is not relieved and circulation restored within a few minutes, the cells in the central portion die and an ulcer forms. Weak or debilitated patients may be in a poor nutritional state and have impaired circulation. Thus the ulcers frequently do not heal well and may even require skin grafting.

A circle or "doughnut" ring is an ineffective type of padding to use. Although it does prevent pressure on a specific bony prominence, it restricts circulation to the central area by placing the pressure all around it. In general, it is preferable to distribute weight over as large an area as possible. Sets of radiolucent sponges in various shapes and sizes are available in the radiology department for this purpose (Fig. 3-16).

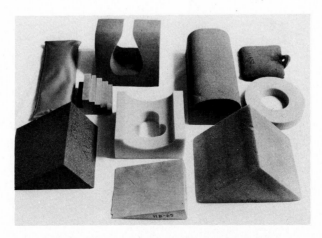

Fig. 3-16. Assortment of positioning aids.

If a patient will be in one position on the x-ray table for longer than 10 minutes, a full-size radiolucent pad should be used. This may be a consideration for debilitated patients undergoing extended studies, such as small bowel series or IV pyelograms for obstructive urinary conditions. If a debilitated patient must be left on the table or on a stretcher for an extended time, the radiographer should assist the patient in changing positions periodically to relieve pressure and maintain circulation.

Positioning is one area in which your learning will be enhanced by acting out the patient role. Practice positioning with your classmates until comfort and positioning are part of the same action.

Skin care

Precautions must be taken to protect the skin while moving and positioning patients. Rough handling or sliding against the table surface may injure the skin of elderly or debilitated patients. When the underlying subcutaneous fat layer is lost, any shear pressure can cause the skin to tear and bleed. The skin of the feet and legs is especially delicate on patients whose circulation is compromised; you must pay special attention to avoid bumping this skin. Even very minor abrasions may increase the likelihood of decubitus ulcer formation. For the same reason, you must keep the patient clean and dry. Patients who perspire heavily or who are incontinent of urine or feces may develop skin irritation that predisposes to ulcer formation.

Safety straps and rails

Safety straps or compression bands may be used on the x-ray table as a precaution against falling. Stretchers are equipped with safety straps or side rails to ensure that patients will not fall or attempt to climb off without assistance. This is especially important when the patient's state of consciousness is impaired because of sedation, intoxication, shock, or senility. Application of straps or side rails is such an important safety practice that it is followed without exception (Fig. 3-17).

RESTRAINTS AND IMMOBILIZATION

Patients who are active and disoriented may require physical restraints. Student radiographers sometimes feel uncomfortable about using such measures, especially when patients find them objectionable. It is helpful to remember that their purpose is to aid and protect the patient. Although restraints may be annoying to patients, they are neither painful nor harmful when properly used. Remember that the application of physical restraints to an adult patient requires a physician's order.

For adults, restraints are almost always fitted before the patient comes to the radiology department. They may consist of wrist and ankle bands fastened to the bed or stretcher. The same restraints used by the nursing service may be employed by the radiographer. Restrained patients must never be left alone on a stretcher or an x-ray table. If the radiographer must leave the room, another qualified person must be assigned to attend the patient.

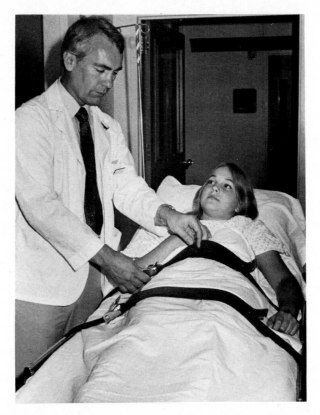

Fig. 3-17. Safety straps or side rails must always be used on stretchers.

It is preferable to win the confidence of small children and to have them submit willingly to examination. Occasionally, however, you must immobilize children for their safety or to meet the procedure's requirements. Fig. 3-18 demonstrates one way to restrain an infant or a small child. Fold down the top edge of a small sheet or lightweight blanket to form an inverted triangle. Place the child supine with shoulders just below the fold. Pull one point of the sheet across one arm, and tuck it behind the back. Then grasp the far point and wrap it around the other arm, once more tucking the end securely under the patient.

Stockinette can be used to immobilize the legs or applied to keep the patient's arms above the head (Fig. 3-19, *A*). There are also infant restraints, such as circumcision boards and various patented devices, that immobilize the child simply and effectively (Fig. 3-19, *B* to *D*).

When patients are coherent and cooperative and are neither sedated nor in distress, the decision to leave the patient alone for a brief period must be based on existing hospital or departmental policy. Many departments have rules that do not allow any patient ever to be left unattended.

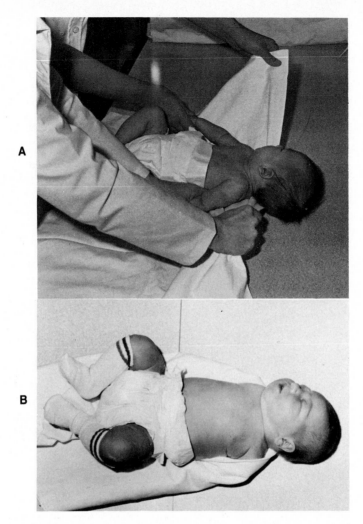

Fig. 3-18. **A,** Small blanket may be used to restrain an infant. **B,** Arms are immobilized with blanket tucked firmly beneath the body.

ACCIDENTS AND INCIDENT REPORTS

Any fall, accident, or occurrence that results in injury or potential harm must be immediately reported to the departmental supervisor. As soon as the victim has been properly attended, one must complete an incident report form. The reporting of incidents is essential whether the victim is a patient, a visitor, or a member of the hospital staff. Do not hesitate to report incidents in which you are injured, even though the injury may seem minor at the time.

Incident reports are crucial to the institution's risk management program. They aid in establishing or limiting the institutional liability for any injury as well as documenting the need for changes that may improve safety practices in

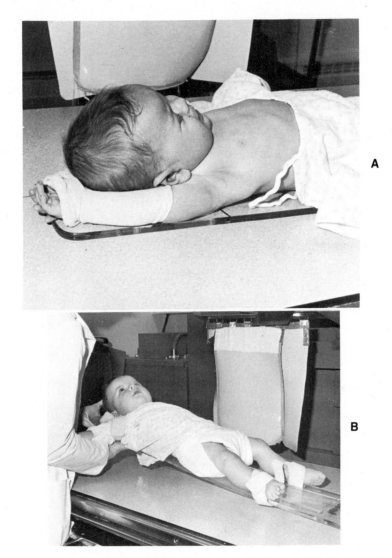

Fig. 3-19. **A,** Stockinette used as a restraining device. **B,** Circumcision board with Velcro straps.   *Continued.*

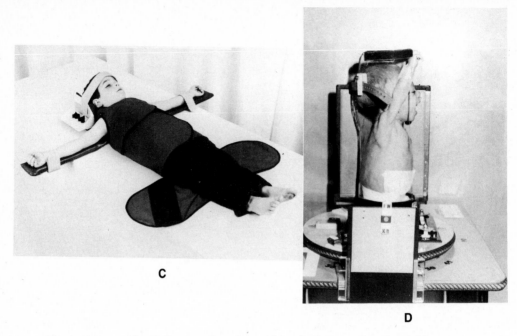

Fig. 3-19—cont'd. C, Papoose Board provides selective restraints for children 2 to 6 years of age. **D,** Pigg-O-Stat infant chair for upright chest radiography. *(Courtesy Olympic Medical, Seattle.)*

the future. Appendix D provides an example of a hospital incident report form. Appendix E contains the safety procedures from a hospital radiology department procedure manual.

CONCLUSION

The principle underlying everything discussed in this chapter is safety. With safety in mind, think before you act, be conscious of hazards, and plan to avoid the occurrence of an accident.

Knowledge of safety rules is indispensable to the radiographer. Whether responding to a fire or moving or positioning a patient on the x-ray table, the objective is to protect patients when they are unable to protect themselves.

Study questions

1. List three appropriate ways to extinguish a limited fire (e.g., in a wastebasket).
2. List four reasons why a patient may *not* be allowed to use the wheelchair for transport or walk to the table in the examination room.
3. Why should specific terms be used to describe the position (in bed or on the examining table) for patients?
4. Why should an incident report be filed even for a minor injury?
5. List three ways in which the principles of good body mechanics can be used at home in the same manner recommended at work.

Evaluating and Meeting Physical Needs

Objectives

At the conclusion of this chapter, the student will be able to:

1. State four reasons for learning good evaluation skills.
2. Demonstrate how to drain and measure the output from a urinary collection bag.
3. List three personal comfort needs common to most patients.
4. Demonstrate how to take a history appropriate to a specific procedure.
5. Find the admitting diagnosis on the patient's chart.
6. Take and record temperature, pulse, and respiration.
7. Obtain and record blood pressure readings.
8. Describe the difference between a carotid and an apical pulse.
9. Use terms such as *dyspneic, diaphoretic,* and *tachycardiac* in describing patients.
10. State the norms for temperature, pulse, respiration, and blood pressure.

Vocabulary list

1. apex, apical
2. atrium
3. bradycardia
4. cyanotic
5. decreased LOC
6. diaphoretic
7. diastolic
8. emesis
9. emphysema
10. feces
11. fibrillation
12. incontinence
13. metabolism
14. NPO
15. qualitative
16. quantitative
17. shock
18. systolic
19. tachycardiac
20. ventricle

Four important reasons exist for the radiographer to develop skills in patient evaluation: (1) to help meet the patient's personal needs, (2) to assist the radiologist by gathering pertinent information, (3) to aid in setting priorities, and (4) to identify changes in the patient's condition that indicate a potential emergency.

MEETING PERSONAL NEEDS

The medical environment intimidates some patients, preventing them from making their physical needs known. The patient who is confident that personal needs will be met is more cooperative and receptive to directions. Personal needs in this context refer to anything the patient requires besides the current procedure's specific demands.

One of the most common and urgent needs is to void, which may cause discomfort and irritability. If this need is ignored in an older or debilitated patient, incontinence may result, causing acute embarrassment for the patient as well as cleanup problems for the radiographer. The radiographer must be especially sensitive to the need for bedpan, urinal, or bathroom facilities when procedures are prolonged.

Be alert to urinary catheters, collection bags, and orders for specimen collection. Occasionally a patient must have a specimen of urine or feces collected. The nursing staff should call this to your attention. Make sure the correct container is available, and ask the nursing staff for instructions if you are unfamiliar with the procedure. Patients sometimes require a quantitative test that demands that *all* specimens be saved, and your failure to comply may invalidate an entire 24-hour urine collection.

When patients are transferred from the wheelchair or stretcher to the radiographic table, the urine collection bag must be held below the level of the patient's bladder. Otherwise, urine in the tube or bag will be siphoned back into the bladder, causing discomfort and allowing bacteria potential access into the bladder.

If the bag is full, it must be emptied, and the urine may need to be measured. Some collection bags consist of a rigid measuring container within a flexible plastic reservoir (Fig. 4-1). Urine flows first into the graduated section. Tipping the unit empties the measured urine into the reservoir. Most collection bags have a drainage outlet at the bottom. Wearing protective gloves, open the stopcock and allow the bag to empty into a waste container or a graduated pitcher, as necessary. *Reclose* the stopcock. Always note the amount emptied, since patients with urinary catheters require fluid intake and output measurement. Record the quantity of urine produced. Note the amount of oral fluid taken *if* oral fluids are allowed.

Anxiety or medication may cause a dry mouth. A drink of water, offered with a straw if the patient cannot sit up, may be very comforting. Before offering fluids to an inpatient, check the chart and note whether oral fluids are permitted. Do not forget to record the amount taken. Often, patients receiving intravenous (IV) therapy are allowed nothing at all by mouth; the abbreviation for this order is *NPO*.* This means no food or liquid, not even ice chips or small sips of water, until the physician orders otherwise.

Occasionally a patient requires a sanitary napkin. Know where these are kept. If a soiled napkin is to be removed, provide a paper bag and place it in the proper can for disposal.

Physical comfort is another personal need. Remember that a thin patient on

---

*From the Latin *nihil pro ora* ("nothing by mouth").

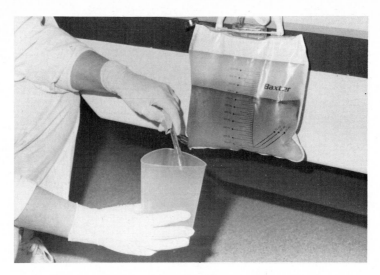

Fig. 4-1. Measuring urinary output.

a hard table will find it difficult to cooperate, especially during a long procedure. Inquire whether the patient is warm enough, and note skin temperature when you touch the patient. As you move about briskly, the room temperature may seem comfortable to you, but elderly or frail patients may not be active enough to keep warm. Use enough blankets, and tuck them in well. This provides both warmth and a sense of reassurance.

Offer tissues to patients who are coughing or sniffling, and position a receptacle within reach for soiled tissues. If dentures or eyeglasses must be removed, place them in a visible, safe location. When you return dentures, rinse them for the patient. They slide in more easily when wet. Glasses, dentures, and hearing aids are essential to patients' activities of daily living and are both difficult and expensive to replace. Choose a safe location for these and similar items, and use it consistently. Purses and other valuables also require a safe location. They may be placed on a counter in full view of the patient. It is helpful to say, "Mr. Garcia, your wallet is right here." This is especially important for outpatients, who are more likely to have these items with them.

The best emotional comfort measure is your presence. Touch patients, and tell them what is to occur. Let them know when you leave the area and when you will return. Escort ambulatory patients to the bathroom or back to their dressing room. It is most distressing for the patient to wander about in a hospital gown, wondering where to go. Once you start a procedure, try to remain with the patient. Postpone your lunch or break until the procedure is complete. If you must leave and another radiographer takes your place, introduce your substitute and excuse yourself rather than simply vanishing. If patients must wait in a room or dressing room, let them know that you are within hearing distance and that they may call on you for help. A call button is available in most patient bathrooms. Show patients how to use it, and assure them that someone will assist them promptly if they call.

TAKING A HISTORY

Radiologists depend on radiographers to assist them by obtaining accurate information about the patient's history and present condition. The answers you receive from the patient may influence how the examination is conducted. The history also aids the radiologist in focusing the interpretation to meet the referring physician's needs. This does not mean a detailed medical history, but rather a thoughtful consideration of why this particular radiographic study is being done. This is especially important when the request or order does not indicate the attending physician's rationale for ordering the procedure. Most departments have policies stating that such information must be provided, but in practice the information received is often simply the admitting diagnosis, which may seem completely irrelevant without explanatory information.

The information you obtain may depend on your ability to gain the patient's confidence. Do not try to obtain clinical information before you have introduced yourself, identified the patient, and responded to any immediate patient needs. Begin by asking a general question about the nature of the problem, such as, "Do you know why Dr. Chen wants you to have an x-ray of your chest?" or "How did you injure your wrist?" The answer to your first question provides clues on how to proceed. The area to be radiographed is stated on the requisition and helps you to focus your query. The questions in Table 4-1 provide a guide for obtaining a history according to the nature of the examination or the body part involved.

Tact and caution are required when obtaining a history. Anxious patients may interpret your questions as suggestions of threatening possibilities. Information regarding such serious matters as cancer, surgery, or heart attack are best elicited in a general way rather than through blunt questions. "Do you know why your doctor ordered this examination?" is less threatening than "Is your doctor checking for cancer?"

If your patient's initial responses are vague, you may need to elicit more specific information. Assuming a negative response can be a helpful way to approach a sensitive subject for the first time, "You haven't been having any heart problems, have you?" is preferable to "Have you ever had a heart problem before?"

Certain examinations require very specific histories, and the exact information required varies among radiologists. You can often meet these requirements by asking the patient to complete a questionnaire before the study. If IV iodine contrast is to be given, your history will also include allergy information and any available data on the patient's renal function (see Chapter 9).

Examinations for patients with chronic conditions or those receiving post-treatment follow-up may require a comparison to prior diagnostic examinations. If these are not part of the current file, your history should include information on previous relevant examinations and when and where they were done.

Record your history briefly on the proper form. Table 4-1 includes examples of history information taken by radiographers.

At this point, the process of taking a history may seem complex and confusing. This is a skill that improves with practice. Role playing with other students,

Table 4-1

Guidelines for taking a history

Examination	Questions	Observations	Example of history*
Orthopedic, acute injury	How did the injury occur? When? Can you show me exactly where it hurts?	Swelling Deformity Discoloration Laceration Abrasion	Twisting injury while skiing today; swelling & pain over lateral malleolus.
Orthopedic, not involving acute injury	Where does it hurt? How long has it been bothering you? Were you ever injured there? How was the injury treated? (Cast? Surgery?) Has there been any recent change?	Deformity Range of motion Weight bearing	Chronic pain × 2 yrs, worse since building fence Sat. Prev Rx c̄ cortisone inj. No known injury.
Neck	Did you injure your neck? How? When? Where does it hurt? Do you have any pain, numbness, or tingling of the shoulder or arm? Which side?		MVA 10/12/92; lt lower neck pain & lt shldr pain c̄ numbness & tingling, lt hand, × 1 mo.
Spine	Did you injure your back? How? When? Do you have pain, numbness, tingling, or weakness of the hip or leg? Which side? Any bowel or bladder problems?		Lifting injury 2 wks ago. LBP radiating to rt hip.
Head	Were you injured? How? Do you have pain? Where? Have you lost consciousness? For how long?	Speech Orientation Gait normal?	Severe HA, blurred vision, dizziness, & gen'l weakness × 24 hrs. No known injury. Speech slurred.
Chest	Do you know why your doctor ordered this examination? Are you short of breath? Do you have a cough? Do you cough anything up? Do you cough up blood? Have you had a fever? Do you have any heart problems?	Respirations Cough	SOB, wheezing, & rt chest pain since resp flu 4 wks ago. Moderate, nonproductive cough.

*Can you identify the common abbreviations used by radiographers (e.g., MVA, motor vehicle accident)? See Appendix C.   *Continued.*

Table 4-1

Guidelines for taking a history—cont'd

Examination	Questions	Observations	Example of history*
Abdomen, gastrointestinal examinations	Do you know why your doctor ordered this examination? Do you have pain? Where? Do you have nausea? Diarrhea? Have you had any other tests for this problem? (Lab tests? Ultrasound?) Do you know the results? Have you ever had abdominal surgery? When? Why?		LLQ pain, incr over past mo. ? of mass seen on US done here 10/21/92.
Urology	Do you know why your doctor ordered this examination? Do you have pain? Where? For how long? Do you have trouble passing urine? Pain? Urgency? Frequency? Have you ever had this problem before? Do you have high blood pressure?		2 prior episodes of UTI; current malaise, fever, & mid back pain.

including a critical observer, will improve your ability so that you can take a patient's history with confidence. As clinical practice provides additional knowledge and experience, you will find that your observation and history skills become increasingly accurate and pertinent.

ASSESSING STATUS

Checking the chart

The radiographer is often required to evaluate the patient's current status. To do this effectively, you can use several available aids. It is important to review the chart or outpatient requisition before you start the procedure. If you have access to an inpatient chart, read the admitting diagnosis and the most recent progress notes and orders. An order for the radiographic procedure should be there. A survey of the current progress notes helps you to assess the patient's physical state and determine whether the preparation for the examination has been done successfully. The nurses' notes may also be helpful. If a recent notation reads, "Unable to stand to void," you can anticipate a need for help when transferring this patient to the x-ray table. A statement such as "emesis × 3" in the nurses' notes just before the examination should be brought to the radiologist's attention *before* proceeding with a barium swallow. Medication may be needed to calm the patient's stomach or nerves long enough for the examination to be completed. If such medication has already been given, it may affect the patient's peristaltic action and therefore the radiologist's interpretation of the fluoroscopic study. Some notations have special significance to the radiographer. Allergies are noted in red, usually on the outside of the chart holder as well as in the history. A patient with a previous history of allergies, sometimes referred to as an "allergenic" individual, is more likely to have an adverse reaction to contrast media. Therefore a complete account of allergies must be reported to the radiologist if the patient is to receive contrast media for the examination. Further assessment of allergy potential is discussed in Chapter 9. Patients in critical condition are usually assigned to the intensive care unit, and their x-ray examinations are done using mobile units (see Chapter 10). Those who must come to the radiology department are usually accompanied by a nurse or a physician.

Setting priorities

An often neglected aspect of patient assessment is the need to set priorities. Radiographers frequently schedule the operation of a specific room and may be responsible for sequencing patients efficiently. Good evaluation skills allow you to be flexible in arranging the schedule to meet the needs of patients who are acutely ill, are obviously in pain, or present valid emergencies and also allow you to feel comfortable while you do it.

Physical signs

How do you know when the patient's condition is changing for the worse? What do you look for? The most important process is typically known as "eyeballing the patient." This skill of acute observation compares the actions and appearance of *this* patient with those of similar patients you have seen. You can also use this skill to compare the appearance of this patient *now* with his or her appearance earlier. Although it may seem intuitive, you actually respond to subliminal changes in the patient's overall appearance or attitude. It takes only an instant to use these skills and to look closely at patients as you admit them to the room.

One of the easiest signs to recognize is *skin color*. Individual complexions vary, but when pale skin becomes cyanotic or olive skin takes on a waxen pallor, the change is apparent. Any patient who looks pale and anxious and says, "I don't feel well," needs to lie down immediately. A patient who loses consciousness and falls to the floor may suffer injuries more serious than the cause of the fainting.

The term *cyanotic* describes a bluish coloration in the skin and indicates a lack of sufficient oxygen in the tissues. This is most easily seen on mucous membranes, such as the lips or the lining of the mouth. Nail beds may also show a bluish tinge. For some patients with heart or lung conditions, this may be a chronic or usual state, but a patient who *becomes* cyanotic needs oxygen and immediate medical attention.

We have discussed the importance of touch as a form of communication and reassurance, but touching also allows you to make direct observations. The acutely ill patient in pain may be pale, cool, and *diaphoretic,* in what is frequently called a "cold sweat." Hot, dry skin may indicate a fever. Warm, moist skin might be a response to a warm room or may indicate acute anxiety. Wet palms and shaking hands are typical of the apprehensive individual who may need an unusual amount of reassurance and whose ability to comprehend and to follow instructions may be seriously impaired. If you note any of these signs, you next need to determine whether this is a new symptom. Has the patient just received an injection of contrast medium or a new medication? If so, notify your supervisor or the radiologist immediately.

Vital signs

The next four procedures used for assessment are usually referred to as vital signs. They involve the measurement of temperature, pulse rate, respiratory rate, and blood pressure. Radiographers do not take vital signs on most patients, but when the need does arise, it is often in response to an urgent situation. The patient in anaphylactic shock does not need a radiographer who wonders whether there is a right or wrong side to a blood pressure cuff! Sharpen your skills at taking vital signs before using them on patients, and review your technique frequently. During slow afternoons, check each other and the receptionist as well. We should all know our own baseline vital signs, so practice will benefit you, the person on whom you practice, and the patient who needs your skill in an emergency.

Most radiology departments have a drawer or box in which are kept a blood pressure cuff and gauge (sphygmomanometer), a stethoscope, and other equipment that might be needed in an emergency. Know where this equipment is stored. Even before you are proficient in its use, you may be asked to obtain it for a physician.

Temperature.   The first of the vital signs is temperature. Although you will have few occasions to check a patient's temperature, it is part of your general professional ability to be able to do so. In addition, this skill can be used in your own home. Body temperature is a measurement of the body's metabolic state. Fever is the sign of an increase in body metabolism, usually in response to an infectious process. Body temperatures vary during the day and are lowest in the early morning and highest in the evening. Normal oral temperatures vary from 98° to 99° F (37° C). Rectal temperatures range from 0.5 to 1.0° higher than oral temperatures, and axillary temperatures range from 0.5 to 1.0° lower. In addition, normal temperatures vary slightly from person to person. A tense, "high-strung," quick-moving individual is likely to have a higher basic temperature than the placid, slow-moving individual, all else being equal. What is your average temperature range?

Temperatures may be taken orally, rectally, or in the axilla. Alert, coopera-

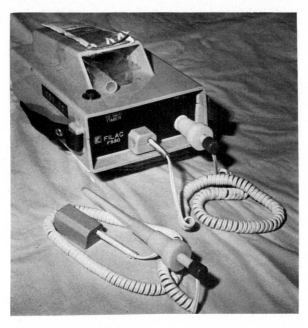

Fig. 4-2.   Electronic digital thermometer is accurate and saves time.

tive individuals usually prefer the familiar oral route. It has long been held that the oral method is less accurate than the rectal method, but recent research does not confirm this belief. The oral method has been shown to provide an accurate measure of changes in body core temperature when taken correctly with the thermometer's bulb well under the base of the tongue.

The oral method is *not* appropriate when the patient has recently drunk hot or cold beverages, is on oxygen, or must breathe through the mouth. In these situations the rectal or axillary method may be used. The rectal temperature is accurate and faster, whereas the axillary temperature is slower and somewhat less accurate. The axillary method is sometimes preferred, however, because it is less invasive. Rectal temperatures may also be contraindicated in certain patients with cardiac conditions to avoid the chance of stimulating the vagus nerve.

Most hospitals now use digital electronic thermometers (Fig. 4-2) on patient care units. These instruments can be read in 1 minute or less. They have disposable sleeves to cover the probe, which avoids the need to disinfect the thermometer after each use. Several types of digital thermometers are available, but in general the following rules apply to all types.

⟶ Taking a patient's temperature

Digital thermometer
1. Wash your hands, and put on disposable gloves.
2. Cover the probe with a clean plastic sleeve.
3. Actuate the thermometer, and insert the probe under the tongue.

4. Remove probe when the audible tone or flashing number indicates that the maximum temperature has been reached (about 1 minute).
5. Note the temperature, and remove plastic sleeve.
6. Remove and discard gloves.
7. Make sure thermometer is off, and return to storage.
8. Record the temperature.

Since you may not have access to a digital thermometer, we have also included directions for glass thermometers.

Glass thermometers may be kept dry or in an antiseptic solution and may be stored in containers labeled "oral" or "rectal." The rectal thermometer sometimes has a shorter, more rounded bulb but is otherwise the same as the oral thermometer.

⏩ Glass thermometer

Oral
1. Wash your hands.
2. Rinse the thermometer if it is stored in antiseptic liquid.
3. Hold the thermometer firmly by the top, and briskly shake the mercury down to 96° F.
4. Place the thermometer bulb under the patient's tongue and leave it in place a minimum of 3 minutes.
5. Remove and read the thermometer.
6. Cleanse the thermometer and return it to be sterilized using the current procedure in your clinical area.
7. Wash your hands and record results.

Axillary
1. Wash your hands.
2. Obtain an oral thermometer (the longer bulb exposes more mercury to body heat).
3. Shake the mercury down to 96° F.
4. Explain to the patient what you are about to do.
5. Place the thermometer bulb into the axilla so that skin folds are in direct contact with bulb.
6. Instruct the patient or hold upper arm firmly to chest wall for 5 to 7 minutes.
7. Remove and read the thermometer.
8. Return the thermometer to be sterilized.
9. Wash your hands and record results.

Rectal
1. Wash your hands. Don gloves.
2. Obtain a rectal thermometer. Its shape may be the same as that of an oral thermometer, but the color on the top is red for rectal.
3. Shake the mercury down to 96° F.
4. Obtain a water-soluble lubricant and apply to the bulb. Have tissues at hand.
5. Explain to the patient what you are going to do.

6. Instruct the patient to lie in a lateral recumbent position. Cover the patient, and expose the anus by raising the top fold of the buttock.
7. Slowly insert the bulb until the anal sphincter is passed, and hold in place for 3 minutes. *Do not leave the patient.*
8. Remove the thermometer slowly. Wipe it with a tissue and read.
9. Cleanse the thermometer, and return it to be disinfected.
10. Remove gloves; wash your hands and record results.

Remember: *always* tell your patient what you are about to do. Place the oral thermometer under the tongue for no less than 3 minutes, preferably for 5 minutes. Remind patients not to bite down and to keep their lips closed.

Most hospitals specify rectal or axillary temperatures for children under the age of 6 years and for anyone who is confused or unable to follow directions. Never leave a patient alone with a rectal or axillary thermometer in place.

Comatose patients in the intensive care unit (ICU) and patients in the neonatal ICU who have unstable body temperatures can now be monitored continuously by using a probe inserted in the external ear canal. A digital readout monitors values. Disposable thermometers are also available (Fig. 4-3). Some disposable thermometers consist of a strip of temperature-sensitive paper with adhesive backing that may be attached to a child's forehead.

Pulse. Counting a pulse rate is such a familiar task to many health professionals that they do it almost automatically and note variations from normal immediately. A pulse is the advancing pressure wave in an artery caused by the ex-

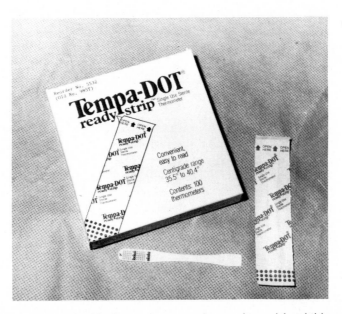

Fig. 4-3. Disposable thermometers are frequently used for children.

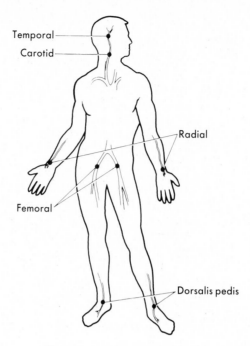

Fig. 4-4. Common pulse points.

pulsion of blood when the left ventricle of the heart contracts. Since this wave occurs with each contraction of the ventricle, it is an easy and effective way to measure the rate at which the heart is beating. A rapid pulse (called *tachycardia* when more than 100 beats/minute) may result from excitement, exertion, or a damaged heart. A rapid pulse rate may also indicate interference with oxygen supply or loss of blood. This results because the heart must beat faster to circulate the remaining blood and carry as much oxygen as possible to the cells. An extremely slow heart rate, or *bradycardia* (less than 60 beats/minute), may indicate that an individual is very athletic or that the heart has a nerve conduction defect. In addition to rate, the pulse volume or quality may vary. A weak or "thready" pulse, especially if the rate is quite rapid, may indicate that a heart is not pumping enough blood.

Common pulse points are shown in Fig. 4-4. The most frequent site for palpation of the pulse is the radial artery at the base of either thumb. Since your own thumb has a pulse, place three fingers over the artery with your thumb on the back of the wrist. Compress gently but firmly. By compressing the artery against the radius, the pulse is easy to feel, especially if the patient's wrist is held palm down (Fig. 4-5).

If the pulse is difficult to count or is weak, you can use the carotid artery. Place your fingers just below the angle of the mandible (Fig. 4-6). The site is easily accessible and is particularly important if a patient loses consciousness. If the pulse is not palpable at this site, the heart is not beating effectively and emergency measures are necessary (see Chapter 7).

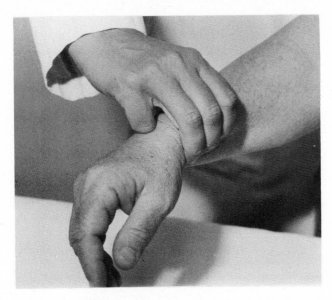

Fig. 4-5. Taking a radial pulse with patient's palm down.

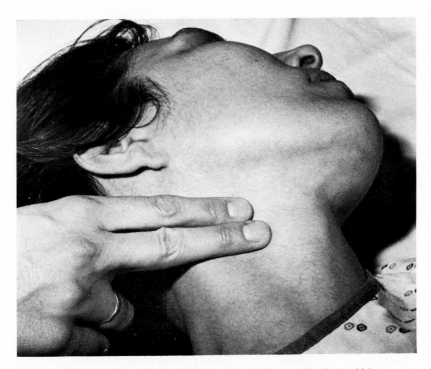

Fig. 4-6. Palpate for carotid pulse just below angle of mandible.

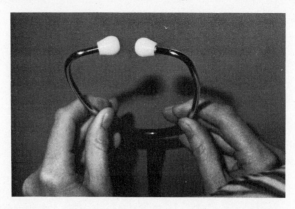

Fig. 4-7. Correctly placed ear tips improve accuracy when using a stethoscope.

If the radial pulse is slow or irregular, you may want to use a stethoscope to take an apical pulse. Look at the stethoscope carefully and become familiar with its use. It may have a bell as well as a diaphragm, although the inexpensive models may have a diaphragm only. On the bimodal stethoscope, you can switch from one mode to the other. For most purposes the diaphragm is preferred. Hold the earpieces of the stethoscope horizontally in front of you (Fig. 4-7). The ear tips should point up slightly. Insert the tips and then tap the diaphragm gently with your finger to be sure you can hear. Now press the diaphragm firmly over the heart's apex, or tip. This is normally found in the fifth anterior intercostal space at the midclavicular line. Count the pulse for a full minute and record the rate and any irregularities. When the apical rate is faster than the radial rate, the heart is not beating efficiently. Inform the physician of this immediately.

Mrs. Nelson, age 70, felt "a bit lightheaded" when she sat up after her IV pyelogram. Her pulse rate is 110. Should you be alarmed? Is this a normal rate for her?

Look in the chart for Mrs. Nelson's previous rates. If she has atrial fibrillation, her resting pulse may be quite rapid. On this occasion, she sat quietly for a minute, and the lightheaded feeling passed. She may have had transient postural or orthostatic hypotension. If such an episode persists, the patient should lie down while the pulse and blood pressure are checked. Any chest pain accompanied by diaphoresis and an increase in pulse rate should be called to the physician's attention immediately.

A pulse oximeter is a digital monitor connected to the patient by means of a cable and a small probe attached to a finger (Fig. 4-8). The readout provides continuous reporting of the heart rate and the oxygen saturation of the blood expressed as a percentage. Pulse oximeters are used during diagnostic imaging studies, particularly magnetic resonance imaging (MRI), to monitor pulse and respiration of patients who must be sedated.

Respirations.   When assessing a patient, do not overlook the respiratory rate. You should inform the radiologist of any difficult breathing *(dyspnea)* or rapid breathing *(tachypnea)* and prepare oxygen apparatus for use.

Whenever a patient shows evidence of respiratory distress, the respiratory rate helps in accurate assessment of the problem. To count respirations, simply note the numbers of inhalations per minute. This is done while continuing to hold the wrist after the pulse has been counted, since some patients may force a change in rate if aware that a count is being made. If you are having difficulty counting breaths, place one hand lightly on the patient's diaphragm. Compare your findings with a normal rate of 12 to 16 breaths/minute.

Not all patients with breathing difficulties need oxygen at a high rate of flow. A patient with pulmonary emphysema or chronic obstructive pulmonary disease (COPD) requires a low flow rate (2 to 3 L/minute), which will provide additional oxygen but will not depress or slow respirations. When patients with emphysema come to the radiology department, check their chart to find out if emphysema is their presenting condition (the problem that brings them to the hospital). Frequently the emphysematous patient who needs a hernia repair or other surgery comes in for an evaluation before admission. Patients with pulmonary emphysema share several characteristics. An increased anteroposterior diameter gives them a barrel-chested appearance. This is frequently associated with an elevation of the shoulder girdle and retraction of the neck muscles, symptomatic of costal respirations. If these patients have received instruction in positive-pressure breathing, you will observe that they purse their lips when exhaling. Recognition of the emphysematous patient is a valuable skill from a technical viewpoint as well, since these patients require special adjustments in exposure for chest radiography.

Another problem with respiration involves the anxious, tense individual who breathes too deeply too often (hyperventilates) and then feels faint or dizzy or complains of tingling and numbness in the extremities. These patients have breathed in too much oxygen and have lost too much carbon dioxide, which disturbs the blood's chemical balance. Try to persuade them to breathe more

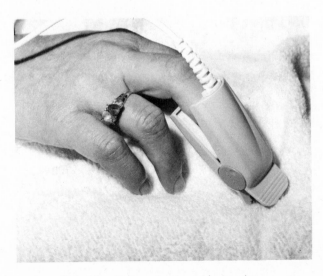

Fig. 4-8. Pulse oximeter probe in place.

slowly or to breathe in and out into a paper bag, which will help return the carbon dioxide level of their blood to normal.

Patients in shock or with significant blood loss have a marked increase in pulse rate and in rapid, shallow breathing as the body attempts to supply oxygen to the tissues by increasing the speed of circulation. Pleurisy or abdominal pain may also cause rapid, shallow breathing as the patient attempts to avoid pain by moving the affected area as little as possible.

Remember that patients with pulmonary disease should not be forced to lie flat if this makes them feel at all short of breath. When lying flat, the weight of the abdomen and abdominal organs pushes against the diaphragm. Patients who are already having difficulty breathing may find this acutely uncomfortable.

> Mr. Widener is going to have a lumbar spine examination. His 30 years of heavy smoking have taken their toll, and while you are positioning him on the table, he becomes short of breath and terribly anxious. What should you do?

The first action is always to help the patient to a more comfortable position. An upright position may enable the patient to breathe easier. Count the pulse rate and respirations. Has there been a change in skin color? Is there evidence of diaphoresis or pain? If your assessment shows cause for concern, notify your supervisor or the radiologist.

Blood pressure.   A blood pressure recording is usually expressed in two figures, such as $^{120}/_{78}$. The top figure (systolic) is a measure of the pumping action of the heart muscle itself. The diastolic pressure* indicates the arterial system's ability to accept the pulse of blood forced into the system by the left ventricle's contraction. If you are angry, afraid, or exercising, the top figure greatly increases. The diastolic figure may also rise, but probably to a lesser degree. What is a *normal* blood pressure? Many figures are used, but as a rule of thumb, an average diastolic pressure greater than 90 mm Hg indicates some degree of hypertension. Less than 50 mm Hg may indicate shock. Blood pressures of $^{100}/_{60}$ to $^{148}/_{88}$ might be considered an acceptable range, depending on age, weight, and physical status.

Although sphygmomanometers are usually used to measure blood pressure in the radiology department, you may observe that some patients are monitored by means of a blood pressure cuff with continuous digital readout. A cuff is placed around the patient's arm, inflates intermittently, and records on a digital readout. This allows the potentially unstable patient to be monitored closely, even when the radiographer is in the control booth. In the ICU you may also observe nurses using a Doppler unit to measure blood pressure when patients have an extremely weak or low pressure.

If an outpatient is to receive IV contrast or systemic medication, it is important to take a blood pressure reading before the procedure begins. Hospital patients will have had a reading recorded but it is advisable to check for this in the chart. Most patients you will see in the radiology department are in stable

---

*An easy way to remember is to think, "D is for down."

Fig. 4-9.

Taking a blood pressure reading.

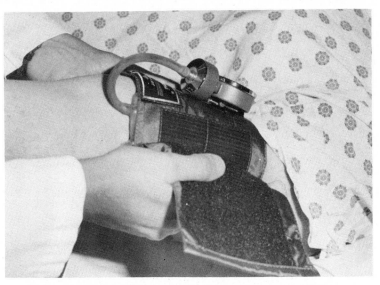

Wrap cuff snugly with bottom of cuff just above antecubital space.

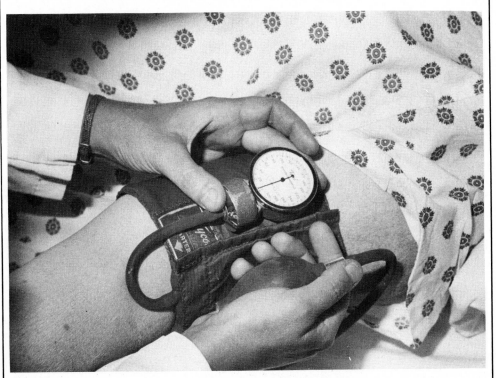

Place gauge for easy visibility of dial.

Continued.

Fig. 4-9.

Taking a blood pressure reading—cont'd.

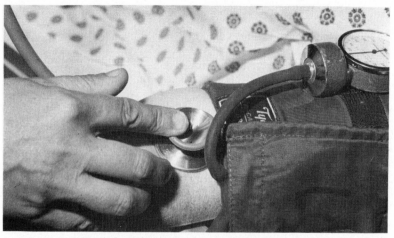

Place stethoscope diaphragm over brachial artery.

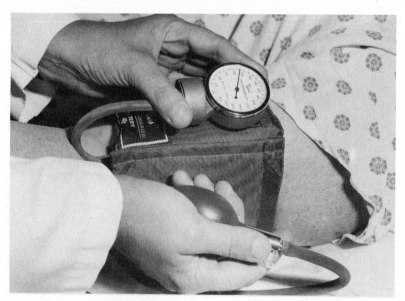

Close pump valve and inflate cuff; release *slowly* to obtain reading.

condition, and blood pressure readings are seldom necessary. The usual reasons for taking a blood pressure reading are to monitor reactions to a drug or contrast medium and to monitor a sudden deterioration in the patient's condition in an emergency or after surgery. Therefore, when you *do* need to measure blood pressure, you must be accurate and must do it quickly. Skills that are used infrequently tend to diminish, so keep your proficiency high by practicing on co-workers, family, or friends. The procedure for taking blood pressure manually is illustrated in Fig. 4-9.

➡ Measuring blood pressure

Wall-mounted or rolling floor-model sphygmomanometers that measure blood pressure in millimeters of mercury (mm Hg) are the most accurate. Small, portable, aneroid manometers are more often found in the radiology department and are sufficient for most purposes.

1. Wash your hands, and explain the procedure to the patient.
2. The patient may be sitting or lying, but the cuff should be at the level of the heart. Either arm can be used.
3. Wrap the cuff snugly with the bottom edge above the antecubital space. Most cuffs are self-securing or fasten with tape.
4. Place the gauge where you can easily read the dial.
5. Palpate the antecubital space for the brachial artery pulse.
6. Place the stethoscope's ear tips in your ears, and press its diaphragm over the brachial artery.
7. Close the valve on the bulb pump, and inflate the cuff rapidly to approximately 180 mm Hg.
8. Open the valve on the pump and release the pressure very slowly.
9. Listen for the beat of the pulse while watching the gauge. Note the figure at which the pulse is first heard. Record this as the systolic reading.
10. As the pressure is released, the sound increases in intensity and then suddenly becomes much softer. Record this point as the diastolic reading.
11. Release the remaining pressure.
12. Have the patient clench and release the fist, and repeat the procedure to check the results.
13. Remove the cuff, and record the results as systolic/diastolic (e.g., $^{140}/_{86}$).
14. Return the equipment to the storage area, and clean the ear tips and diaphragm with alcohol.

You must average three blood pressure readings if you are taking a baseline or average blood pressure. In an emergency, however, you must report your reading immediately to the physician and then compare it with those recorded in the chart. The physician will interpret your reading, but you must be accurate for a valid evaluation of the patient's status to be made.

Now that you are able to observe some pertinent data about your patients, how can you report what you observe? "That guy in B just came unglued" relays feelings of urgency but little else. "Mr. Jones in B has just become diaphoretic, weak, and short of breath and is complaining of substernal pain" is a precise, descriptive statement and gives the physician specific, usable informa-

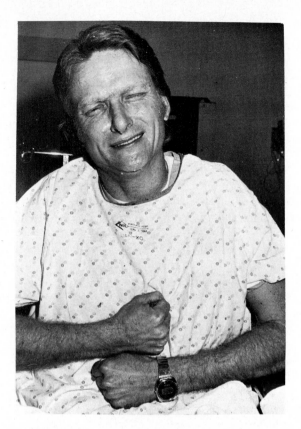

Fig. 4-10. Describe this patient using appropriate terminology (see Appendix C).

tion. One of the best ways to learn the use of descriptive terminology is to use it frequently before an emergency arises. Using the list of terms in Appendix C, describe the patient in Fig. 4-10.

CONCLUSION

The warning words on railway grade crossings in the past read, "Stop, Look, and Listen." These signs were meant to encourage motorists to assess whether it was safe to proceed. The same principle should be applied by the beginning radiographer today: stop, look, and listen to assess the situation before you proceed with patient care.

If you are in doubt about the change in a patient's status, you have resources available to help you, such as your supervisor, the physician, the chart, and the nursing staff.

Stop periodically and think of yourself as an extension of the radiologist and as a patient advocate. *Look* for changes in patients' mental and physical status, and be ready to take steps to avoid emergencies. *Listen* to patients, and meet their needs whenever possible.

Incidentally, the young man in Fig. 4-10 is pale and diaphoretic. His facial expression (grimacing), stooped posture, and the position of his clenched fists indicate acute upper abdominal pain.

Study questions

1. List three reasons why a patient brought to the radiology department might have NPO status.
2. When might it be advisable for a patient to know the location of the bathroom before beginning a procedure?
3. List three occasions when a patient's admitting diagnosis might have no direct relationship to the x-ray order.
4. When would a carotid pulse be preferred to a radial pulse? When would an apical pulse be preferred?
5. Why should you be familiar with the patient's blood pressure *before* an IV pyelogram if the patient has no history of allergy?

5

Infection Control

Objectives

At the conclusion of this chapter, the student will be able to:

1. Define medical asepsis, disinfection, and sterilization.
2. List four factors involved when pathogenic organisms are transferred from person to person.
3. State five examples of personal hygiene that help in preventing the spread of infection.
4. Demonstrate techniques for effective handwashing.
5. Describe the correct method of linen disposal using medical asepsis principles.
6. State the dilution and name the agent used for disinfecting radiographic equipment, as recommended by the Centers for Disease Control.
7. Demonstrate steps used in discarding disposable equipment in the clinical area.
8. Contrast isolation techniques for infectious and immunodeficient patients.
9. State the percentage of health care workers infected with HIV through occupational exposure.
10. Demonstrate removal and disposal of gowns, gloves, and masks without breaking isolation principles.

Vocabulary list

1. asepsis
2. autoclave
3. catheterization
4. chemotherapy
5. disinfection
6. endemic
7. epidemic
8. fomites
9. immunosuppressant
10. lumbar puncture
11. microbial dilution
12. nosocomial
13. opportunistic infection
14. pathogens
15. spores
16. sterile field
17. sterilization
18. vectors

Hospitals are gathering places for the sick and are focal points for the transmission of infection. Anyone with a health problem is more susceptible to infection, and therefore medical asepsis is of critical importance in patient care.

Medical asepsis deals with reducing the *probability* of infectious organisms being transmitted to a susceptible individual. Any organism in an optimum environment will multiply at a rapid rate.

The healthy human body has the ability to overcome a limited number of infectious organisms. This resistance can be overwhelmed by a massive exposure. On the other hand, a reduced resistance caused by disease or chemotherapy may result in infection after only minimal exposure. Therefore, the fewer organisms to which a patient is exposed, the better the chance that he or she will resist infection. The process of reducing the total number of organisms is called *microbial dilution* and can be accomplished at several levels.

Simple *cleanliness* measures avoid transmitting organisms when proper cleaning, dusting, linen handling, and handwashing techniques are used. The second level is *disinfection* and involves the destruction of pathogens by using chemical materials. The third stage is surgical asepsis, or *sterilization*. This involves treating items with heat, gas, or chemicals to make them germ free. They are then stored in a manner that prevents contamination.

CYCLE OF INFECTION

The four factors involved in the spread of disease are sometimes called the cycle of infection (Fig. 5-1). For infections to be transmitted, there must be an infectious organism, a reservoir of infection, a susceptible host, and a means of transporting the organism from the reservoir to the susceptible individual.

Infectious organisms

Infectious organisms are too small to be seen with the naked eye and are referred to as *microorganisms*. They include bacteria, viruses, protozoa, and fungi. Organisms capable of causing disease are called pathogenic organisms, or *patho-*

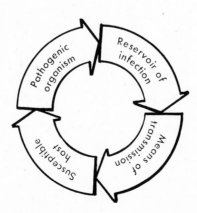

Fig. 5-1. Cycle of infection.

Table 5-1

Some examples of pathogens

System	Name	Classification	Disease	Mode of transmission
Respiratory tract	Bordetella pertussis	Bacterium	Whooping cough	Airborne
	Candida albicans	Fungus	Pneumonia, thrush in infants	Airborne Airborne
	Corynebacterium diphtheriae	Bacterium	Diphtheria	
	Mycobacterium tuberculosis	Bacterium	Tuberculosis	Airborne and droplets
	Mumps virus	Virus	Mumps	Airborne
	Streptococcus pneumoniae	Bacterium	Pneumonia, sinus infections	Airborne
	Streptococcus pyogenes	Bacterium	Strep throat	Airborne
Gastrointestinal tract	Entamoeba histolytica	Protozoan	Amebic dysentery	Food and water
	Giardia lambla	Protozoan	Giardiasis	Food and water
	Poliomyelitis virus	Virus	Poliomyelitis	Food and water
	Salmonella species	Bacterium	Salmonellosis (food infection)	Food and water
	Shigella species	Bacterium	Shigellosis (bacillary dysentery)	Food and water
Genitourinary tract	Escherichia coli	Bacterium	Cystitis, nephritis	Contact
	Herpes simplex, type 2	Virus	Genital herpes	Sexual contact
	Neisseria gonorrhoeae	Bacterium	Gonorrhea	Sexual contact
	Proteus species	Bacterium	Cystitis, nephritis	Contact
	Treponema pallidum	Bacterium	Syphilis	Sexual contact
	Trichomonas vaginalis	Protozoan	Vaginitis	Sexual contact
Skin	Herpes simplex, type 1	Virus	Fever blisters	Contact (and predisposition)
	Measles virus	Virus	Measles	Airborne, contact
	Staphylococcus aureus	Bacterium	Boils, wound infections	Contact
	Tinea capitis	Fungus	Ringworm	Contact (and predisposition)
	Tinea pedis	Fungus	Athlete's foot	Contact (and predisposition)
Blood	Leptospira	Bacterium	Leptospirosis	Food and water
	Plasmodium species	Sporozoan	Malaria	Vectors (mosquitoes)
	Salmonella typhi	Bacterium	Typhoid fever	Food and water

gens. Some microorganisms live on or within the body as part of our normal flora. They aid in digestion and skin preservation and are nonpathogenic as long as they are confined to their usual environment. For example, *Candida albicans* may be found in the throat or gastrointestinal (GI) tract of many healthy persons. Yet this organism can assume a pathogenic role, causing urinary and vaginal infections in females and thrush or respiratory diseases in infants and patients with acquired immunodeficiency syndrome (AIDS). Some common pathogens are listed in Table 5-1.

Reservoir of infection

The reservoir, or source, of infection may be any place where pathogens can thrive in sufficient numbers to pose a threat. Such an environment must provide moisture, nutrients, and a suitable temperature, all of which are found in the human body. A source of infection might be the patient with hepatitis, a radiographer with an upper respiratory infection (URI), or a linen handler with staphylococcal boils.

Since some pathogens live in the bodies of healthy individuals without causing apparent disease, a person may be the reservoir for an infectious organism without realizing it. These persons are called *carriers.* Many of us have throat cultures that are positive for *Staphylococcus aureus,* but we do not have a sore throat. A susceptible patient with an open wound could contract a life-threatening infection if sufficiently contaminated with this organism. The classic example of a carrier of infection is Typhoid Mary, a "healthy" food handler. Hundreds of cases of typhoid fever were attributed to contamination of the meals she helped to prepare. Better sanitation and food-handling education have reduced the incidence of food-borne diseases. Today an example of a carrier of infection is the asymptomatic individual infected with human immunodeficiency virus (HIV) who spreads the disease through sexual intercourse or by sharing contaminated needles with intravenous drug users (IDUs).

Although the human body is the most common reservoir of infection, any environment that will support the growth of microorganisms has the potential to be a secondary source. Such sources include contaminated food or water or any damp, warm place that is not cleaned regularly.

Susceptible host

Susceptible hosts are frequently patients who have a reduced natural resistance to infection. In addition to the primary problem that caused their hospitalization, they may develop a secondary or *nosocomial* (hospital-acquired) infection. Approximately 5% of patients admitted to hospitals each year acquire nosocomial infections. Although many of these infections are non-life-threatening, recent statistics indicate that 20,000 patients a year die of hospital-acquired infections and that more than half of these are preventable. Mr. Fairbrother, a postsurgical patient with a urinary tract infection (UTI), or Mrs. Stuart, a patient with heart disease and a URI, may have acquired such nosocomial diseases.

Hospital-acquired infections also pose a threat to health care workers. In the United States, 8000 to 12,000 health care workers are infected with the hepatitis B virus (HBV) each year, resulting in 200 deaths. This particular strain of hepatitis is highly infectious, requires intensive treatment, and may lead to life-long health problems. In December 1991 the Occupational Safety and Health Administration (OSHA) published regulations that require health care employers to provide HBV immunizations to employees, as well as procedures and equipment to prevent the transmission of HIV and other blood-borne diseases to which employees are exposed.

Hospital workers are exposed to many pathogens (Fig. 5-2). In a single day a radiographer may care for ambulatory outpatients, hospital patients in isolation, and emergency trauma patients with "dirty" wounds. The radiographer who works when his or her resistance is low because of fatigue, stress, or a low-grade infection has become a susceptible host.

Transmission of disease

The most direct way to intervene in the cycle of infection is to prevent transmission of the infectious organism from the reservoir to the susceptible host. To accomplish this successfully, one must understand the four main routes of transmission.

The first route is by means of *direct contact*. This implies that the host is touched by an infected person in such a manner that the organisms are placed in direct contact with susceptible tissue. For example, syphilis and HIV (AIDS) infections may be contracted when infectious organisms from the mucous membrane of one individual are placed in direct contact with the mucous membrane of a susceptible host. Also, skin infections often occur among hospital workers because of the frequent contact with patients who have staphylococcal and streptococcal diseases.

The three other principal routes of transmission are *indirect* and involve transport of organisms by means of fomites, vectors, and airborne contamination.

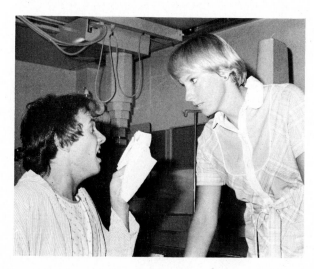

Fig. 5-2. Exposure to infection is a daily hazard to radiographers.

An object that has been in contact with pathogenic organisms is called a *fomite*. The contaminated urinary catheter that caused Mr. Fairbrother's UTI is a good example. Other fomites in the radiology department might include the x-ray table, the calipers, or the radiographer's hands.

A *vector* is an animal in whose body an infectious organism develops or multiplies before becoming infective to a new host. Some examples of vectors are mosquitoes that transmit malaria, fleas that harbor bubonic plague, and animals such as dogs, bats, or squirrels in which rabies is endemic. The bite of infected insects or mammals thus may transmit diseases to humans.

Airborne contamination is spread by means of droplets and dust. Droplet contamination often occurs when an infectious individual coughs, sneezes, or speaks in the vicinity of a susceptible host. Mrs. Stuart, for example, may have acquired her URI from the orderly who sneezed while doing the abdominal preparation.

Although many organisms are fragile, requiring continuous warmth, moisture, and nutriment to exist, others are capable of forming spores. In this stage the organism is resistant to heat, cold, and drying and can live without nourishment. Spores can float through the air and lurk in dusty corners waiting for the opportunity to invade a susceptible host. Spore-forming organisms are responsible for such serious, but relatively uncommon, diseases as tetanus, anthrax, histotoxic infections, gas gangrene, and septicemia. Recent epidemiological studies have shown that some viruses can resist drying for weeks. The viruses that cause herpes (both oral and genital) are examples. This should emphasize to you the need for practical asepsis.

PREVENTING DISEASE TRANSMISSION

At one time, cleanliness was our only defense against infection. We now live in an age that benefits from antibiotics that significantly reduce the suffering and death once caused by infections. However, do not be deluded into thinking that an antibiotic exists for every infectious disease. Viral infections are resistant to most antibiotics. Other organisms, such as staphylococci, apparently mutate rapidly, acquiring immunity against medications that were once highly effective. In any case, disease prevention is clearly preferable to the most efficacious cure. Therefore, the practice of medical asepsis is still the first line of defense in preventing the spread of disease.

Historical perspective

When infectious disease was rampant, infected persons were often "quarantined," which meant that members of a household were prevented from leaving their home and others were excluded to confine the infection to one family rather than spreading it through an entire community. Later, hospitals developed policies that involved separating patients admitted with infectious diseases from other patients. Contacts with other persons were rigidly controlled. This "isolation" was a logical outgrowth of the former practice of quarantine. These techniques provided for specialized methods of asepsis when the danger of disease transmission was exceptionally great.

Although isolation techniques were effective when used correctly, no mechanism existed for the prevention of serious diseases carried by asymptomatic individuals. This has certainly been true of patients who are carriers of HBV and those with HIV, the infectious agent responsible for AIDS.

HIV and AIDS

The rapid spread of HIV infection and AIDS is a source of concern to everyone. Since June 1981, more than 207,000 patients with AIDS have been diagnosed in the United States, and the cumulative AIDS-related deaths is greater than 133,000. Of the estimated 1 million individuals in the United States infected with HIV, approximately 20% have developed AIDS. Since the undiagnosed HIV carrier may be asymptomatic for as long as 10 years, the potential for spreading disease assumes immense proportions. Of the first 100,000 cases reported, 61% occurred among homosexual or bisexual males with no history of being intravenous drug users (IDUs) and 20% among heterosexual male or female IDUs. More recent statistics show a dramatic increase in heterosexual transmission. It is expected that the rate for non-IDU heterosexual transmission will increase 50% by 1995. Although drugs have been developed that prolong the time required for HIV infections to progress to AIDS, at this time no known cure exists. New vaccines have been developed but have not yet been tested and approved for use in the United States.

Fortunately, the AIDS virus is not acquired by casual contact (e.g., touching or shaking hands; eating food prepared by an infected person; contact with drinking fountains, telephones, toilets, or other surfaces). It is not an airborne disease. The routes of transmission are through sexual contact, from contaminated blood or needles, and to the fetus if the mother is infected.

Since AIDS is an immunodeficiency condition, the primary cause of death is a secondary disease or combination of diseases. Among the conditions frequently involved are Kaposi's sarcoma, *Pneumocystis carinii* pneumonia, and other opportunistic infections. One effect of the AIDS epidemic has been a sharp rise in the number of tuberculosis infections. As the incidence of drug-resistant tuberculosis continues to rise, an increasing number of these patients probably will be hospitalized for treatment.

As a health care worker in today's world, you must expect to encounter unidentified or undiagnosed patients with AIDS and HBV. Currently, controversy surrounds the patient's right to confidentiality regarding the AIDS diagnosis, even within the hospital setting. This may prevent you from being informed about diagnosed patients. Also, diagnosed patients are only the "tip of the iceberg." It is estimated that as many as 50 undiagnosed patients with serious viral disease exist for every known case. Anxiety about HIV infections is typical and understandable among health care workers. However, the occupational risk is not great. More than 95% of the health care workers infected with HIV were exposed as a result of activities unrelated to their work. The most common occupational exposure by far is the needle stick. Many thousands of needle sticks have been reported in the last 10 years, but only 41 health care workers with no other identified risk factors have been diagnosed as HIV positive. The implications here are obvious. Although prevention at work is essential, self-care in terms of safe sexual practice is equally crucial.

Universal precautions

Since persons infected with AIDS, HBV, or other diseases (e.g., typhoid fever) may have no symptoms, you must treat all patients as potential reservoirs of infection.

The Centers for Disease Control (CDC) are now recommending a system of infection control called *body substance precautions* (BSP), or universal precautions. This system is based on the use of barriers for all contacts with all body substances rather than focusing on the isolation of a patient with a diagnosed disease. The need to use barriers such as gloves and masks depends on the nature of the interaction with the patient rather than on the specific diagnosis. Emphasis is placed on all body fluids being potential sources of infection, regardless of diagnosis.

Although this system was not developed solely in response to the AIDS epidemic, it does meet all criteria for dealing with these patients, as well as those with other viral diseases and certain bacterial diseases for which no effective antibiotic may exist. Using a BSP program discourages transmission from patient to patient as well as from patient to caregiver. The key to effective protection is a consistent approach to *all* contact with *all* body substances of *all* patients at *all* times.

The information in the box on p. 108 lists recommendations of the CDC. Note that individual judgment is needed in determining when barriers are needed. This means that you will be making frequent decisions about when to take the extra time to protect both yourself and your patients. How you assess these risks and respond to them will vary with the setting and your level of experience. As a beginning student, your level of precaution should be very high. Although you may observe more experienced workers taking fewer precautions, do not think you must follow their example. At this stage in your experience, it is better to take too much precaution rather than too little.

The AIDS epidemic has resulted in much attention given to this topic, and further recommendations may be forthcoming. The hospital or agency where you work will have an infection control department that will incorporate current recommendations into an existing system of isolation and infection control. Be familiar with your institution's current rules.

MEDICAL ASEPSIS

One can easily find examples of poor aseptic technique in most clinical settings. Unfortunately the results of carelessness are seldom traced to the culprit. It is the patient acquiring a nosocomial infection who suffers. Armed with the knowledge of disease transmission, how can you fight the spread of infection?

1. Stay home when you are ill.
2. Cover your mouth when you sneeze or cough.
3. Wear a clean uniform daily, and remove it when you go home.
4. Wash your hands.
5. Use BSP when handling patients, linens, or items contaminated with body substances.
6. Practice good housekeeping techniques.

Body Substance Precautions

1. Wear *gloves* when it is likely that hands will be in contact with body substances (blood, urine, feces, wound drainage, oral secretions, sputum, vomitus).
2. Protect clothing with a plastic *apron* or wear a *gown* when it is likely that clothing will be soiled with body substances.
3. Wear *masks* and/or *eye protection* when it is likely that eyes and/or mucous membranes will be splashed with body substances (e.g., when suctioning a patient with copious secretions).
4. *Wash hands* often and well, paying particular attention to fingernails and the area between the fingers.
5. Discard uncapped needle/syringe units and "SHARPS" in puncture-resistant biohazard containers.
6. If *unanticipated contact* with body substances occurs, wash as soon as possible (handwashing, facewashing, etc., as appropriate).
7. Use gloves to wipe up after *all blood spills,* and disinfect using 1 part bleach to 10 parts water.

Use individual judgment in determining when barriers are needed. Each individual must establish his or her own standards for consistent use of barriers. These personal standards should be based on the individual's skills and interactions with the patient's body substances, nonintact skin, and mucous membranes.

Body substance precautions for all patient care

| Wash hands. | Wear gloves when likely to touch body substances, mucous membranes, or nonintact skin. | Wear plastic apron or a gown when clothing is likely to be soiled. | Wear mask/eye protection when likely to be splashed. | Place intact needle/syringe units and "sharps" in designated disposal container. Do not break or bend needles. |

Handwashing

The first three principles are simple and self-explanatory. Handwashing also may seem obvious, but this is the rule most consistently ignored in many hospital settings. Medically aseptic handwashing technique is both simple and effective. It should be followed explicitly before and after work, before meals, and often during the day. Since a radiographer's duties frequently demand brief contacts with a series of patients, it is especially important that you *always wash your hands between patients* (Fig. 5-3).

| Fig. 5-3. | Handwashing technique. |

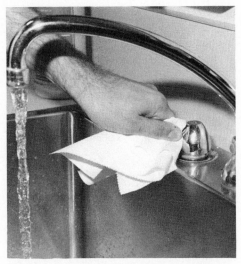

Consider sink to be contaminated and try not to touch it with uniform. Use paper towels to handle controls unless there are foot or knee levers. Adjust water flow to avoid splashing. Adjust temperature for comfort. Allow water to continue running.

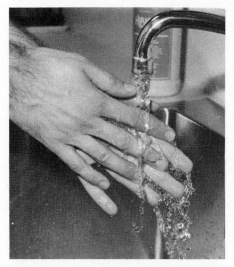

Wet hands thoroughly. Keep hands lower than elbows so water will drain from cleanest area (forearms) to most contaminated area (fingers).

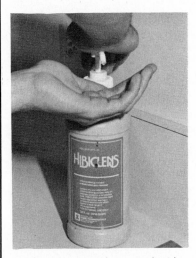

Apply soap. Liquid or powdered soap is preferred. Soap dishes can harbor bacteria and contaminate hands.

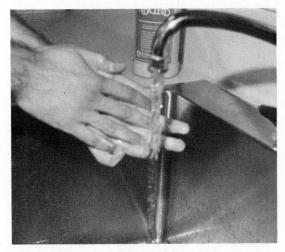

Lather well. Rub hands and fingers together with firm, rotary motion for 20 seconds. (Friction is more effective than soap in removing microorganisms from skin.) Rub palms, areas between fingers, and backs of hands.

Fig. 5-3. **Handwashing technique—cont'd.**

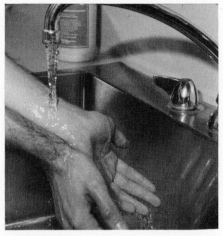

Rinse, allowing water to run down over hands. *Repeat* steps to cleanse wrists and forearms.

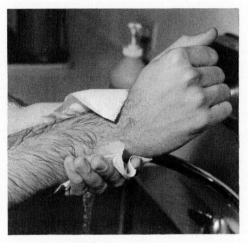

Dry hands thoroughly.

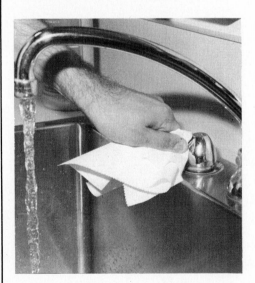

Turn off water with paper towel to avoid contaminating hands.

Good housekeeping also reduces the incidence of airborne infections and the transfer of pathogens by fomites. A clean, dry environment discourages the growth of all microorganisms. Much of the cleaning in the radiology department may be done at night by the housekeeping staff, but the radiographer is responsible for inspecting the work area regularly and maintaining high standards of medical asepsis.

Several general principles apply whenever cleaning is required. Always clean from the least contaminated area toward the more contaminated area and from the top down. Avoid raising dust, and do not contaminate yourself or clean areas.

One of your duties is to clean the radiographic table between patients. Use a cloth moistened with disinfectant such as Cidex, Staphene, Lysol, or Clorox. The CDC recommend sodium hypochlorite bleach (Clorox) as the preferred disinfectant for preventing the spread of HIV. If you use Clorox, you should mix it daily in a 1:10 solution because the effectiveness declines rapidly.

Every piece of equipment that comes in contact with the patient, such as the chest film holder or fluoroscope, must also be cleaned after each use. Most hospitals have written procedures with detailed instructions concerning preferred cleansing agents and the extent of responsibility for disinfecting rooms. Consult the infection control procedure for your clinical area.

Handling linens

Linens may become dangerous fomites if proper aseptic technique is not observed. Objects or linens soiled with body secretions (mucus, vomitus, urine, feces) are considered contaminated, even though stains may not be apparent. Any linens used by patients should be handled as little as possible. To prevent airborne contamination, fold the edges of linens to the middle without shaking or flapping. Immediately place loosely balled linens in the hamper. *Never* use any linen for more than one patient.

You should protect your uniform with a gown while assisting incontinent patients or helping to clean up trauma patients. For the protection of laundry workers, grossly contaminated linens should be placed in a separate plastic bag and marked, for example, "Fecal Contamination" (Fig. 5-4). Many hospitals today provide laundry bags that dissolve in hot water. This reduces the number of times linen must be handled and helps protect the laundry personnel in particular.

The floor in the hospital is always considered grossly contaminated, and anything touching the floor is disposed of immediately. This includes linens as well as instruments and other items. When in doubt as to the cleanliness of any object, do not use it.

Disposal of contaminated waste

A modern hospital uses many disposable items, from simple objects such as paper cups and tissues to more complex items such as catheterization sets. *Disposable items are designed to be used only once and then discarded.* The only exception to this rule involves the immediate reuse of an unsterile item (e.g., emesis basin) by the same patient.

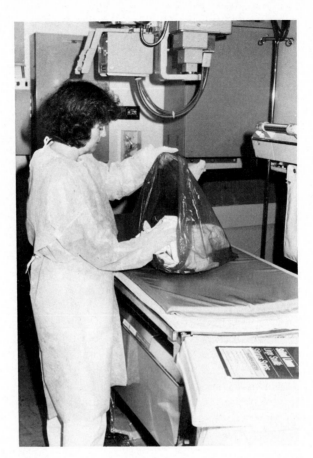

Fig. 5-4. Grossly contaminated linen requires special care.

Each hospital has a routine for the discarding of disposable items. Some separate glass, plastic, and paper into covered containers. Others place everything together. Follow the procedure for your institution. Recent regulations demand that objects contaminated with blood or body fluids be discarded in a suitable container and marked with the biohazard symbol (see Fig. 5-5 for symbol).

Needles and syringes are disposed of in special containers designed to receive the syringe without recapping it with the needle cover (Fig. 5-5). If you *must* recap a syringe (e.g., the container is too far away, or you cannot leave the patient), place the cover on a hard surface and insert the needle without using your other hand (Fig. 5-6). If you frequently need to recap needles, it is helpful to have a needle cap holder attached to the counter in your work area. This holds the cap upright for one-handed needle insertion. Most finger punctures occur while recapping a syringe.

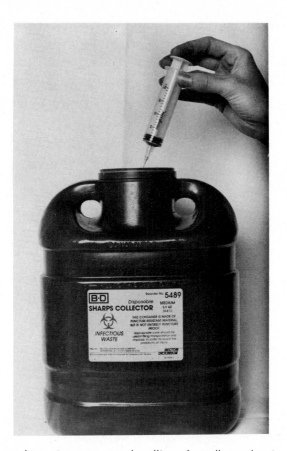

Fig. 5-5. Safe disposal practices prevent rehandling of needles and syringes. Note biohazard symbol.

Be careful not to prick your finger. An accidental needle prick or skin broken by a contaminated object may be cause for concern. If this occurs, an incident report must be filed even though the injury seems insignificant. In addition to an incident report, most hospitals now ask that a baseline blood sample be drawn. Since HIV infection will not be apparent in the blood for approximately 3 months, this helps rule out infection acquired before the occupational exposure. After 3 to 4 months, another blood sample is tested for HIV.

Bandages and dressings should be handled with gloves and should be placed directly into waterproof bags, which should be sealed before discarding.

Always wear gloves when assisting patients with bedpans or urinals. Be sure to empty these at once unless a specimen is needed. Rinse them well over the hopper or toilet, and discard or put them in the proper place to be sterilized unless they are to be reused immediately by the same patient.

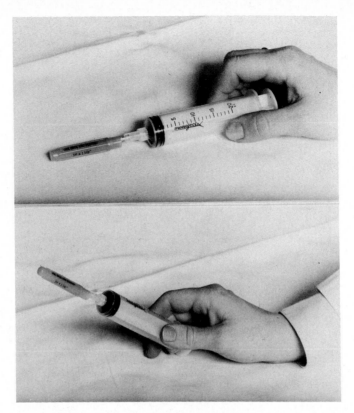

Fig. 5-6. Avoid finger punctures by recapping needles with one hand only.

ISOLATION TECHNIQUE

We recommend that you fully understand and use the BSP procedures previously discussed. Some hospitals have adopted BSP in addition to most of the isolation policies already being used. Isolation may be a requirement for patients with tuberculosis. Therefore, we include a discussion of the various types of isolation.

Formerly the guidelines for isolation precautions in hospitals recommended that each hospital adopt one of two systems for designating the specific precautions required for any isolation situation. Some hospitals may choose to supplement BSP with the *category-specific* system, which identifies seven different types of isolation, depending on the patient's disease or condition. Standard, color-coded cards are placed on the patient's door stating the type of isolation and the specific precautions required. For example, diseases such as influenza, which may be transmitted by airborne droplets, require one to wear a mask and gloves. Diseases that may spread by means of contaminated blood or body fluids (e.g., hepatitis) require one to wear gloves when blood or body fluids are handled. Appendix G summarizes all seven categories according to the precautions recommended and the diseases for which they are appropriate.

The second system of isolation is *disease specific*. That is, the hospital may

Fig. 5-7.

Preparation for examination in strict isolation.

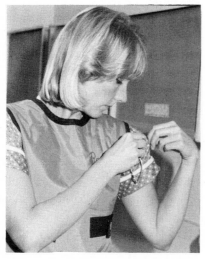

Wearing lead apron, remove jewelry and attach to uniform.

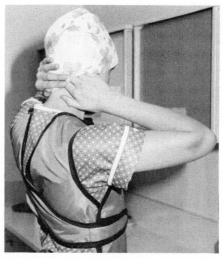

Don cap, making certain that all hair is covered.

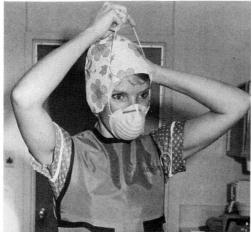

Don mask, making certain nose and mouth are completely covered.

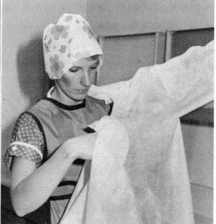

Put on gown.

Continued.

Fig. 5-7.

Preparation for examination in strict isolation—cont'd.

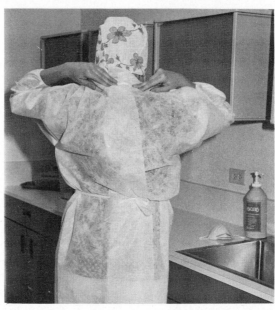

Fasten gown securely with waist tie and neck tape.

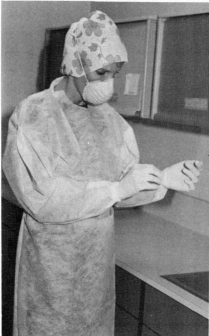

Put on gloves.

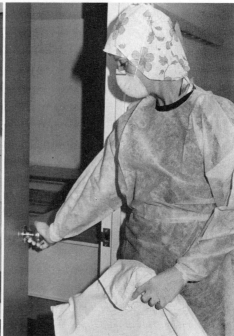

Radiographer approaches patient with cassette in protective cover.

choose to evaluate each case against standard recommendations and use only those precautions that specifically apply. A typical isolation card for use with the disease-specific system is also included in Appendix G.

Patients placed in isolation often tend to feel rejected and "untouchable." You can help alleviate these feelings by expressing a friendly interest in the patient and by avoiding any display of fear or revulsion as you perform your duties.

Radiography of the isolation patient requires two people. The team should consist of two radiographers, one to position the patient and one to handle the equipment. Although both radiographers must follow all designated isolation precautions, one remains "clean" in that he or she has no direct contact with the patient, the bed, or any items the patient may have touched. This radiographer is the only one who handles the x-ray machine and the cassettes. The team method results in the least contamination of x-ray equipment, which is difficult to disinfect completely.

Before entering the isolation room, prepare the necessary cassettes by placing each one in a smooth-fitting plastic bag or pillowcase. Place the mobile x-ray unit inside the room, and don your lead apron. Remove your jewelry and watch, and place them in your pocket or pin them to your uniform. At the door you will find the necessary supplies for the required precautionary measures (e.g., disposable gloves, gowns, masks). Use the posted isolation guidelines for the designated type of isolation, and don protective clothing (Fig. 5-7). If the room was well designed for isolation, this procedure may be done in a vestibule adjoining the patient area.

Now you are ready to approach the bedside. Greet the patient, make introductions, and explain the procedure. Then, wearing gloves, place the cassette under the patient, making certain that the exposure side is facing up (Fig. 5-8). Your teammate will position the machine, set the controls, and make the expo-

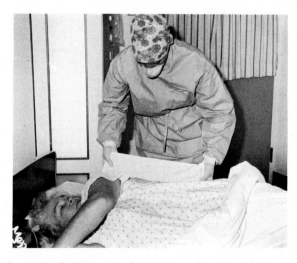

Fig. 5-8. Placing covered cassette under isolation patient.

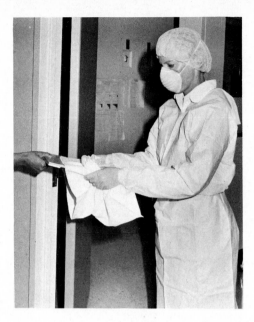

Fig. 5-9. Cassette transfer. Fold back contaminated cover, offering "clean" cassette to teammate.

sure. As each exposure is completed, retrieve the cassette and fold back the cover, offering it to your teammate with the edge exposed (Fig. 5-9). The contaminated cover is then placed in the proper container and the cassette is stored in the machine compartment.

When the examination is completed, make certain that the patient is comfortable and secure. Now, untie your waist belt and remove your gloves. Gloves are removed before taking off the gown. Pull off the first one, gripping it by the contaminated side and inverting it as you remove it. Discard it directly into the container provided. Insert your clean fingers *inside* the cuff of the second glove, once more inverting it as it is removed (Fig. 5-10). Next, untie the neck strings, then the back strings. Remove the mask without touching the face portion; holding it by the strings, place it in the container provided. Now, remove your gown, taking care to hold it away from you; folding the contaminated sides together, place it in the hamper. Wash your hands, remembering to use paper towels to handle the faucets (Fig. 5-11).

Push the mobile x-ray unit outside the room, and clean it thoroughly before taking it back to the radiology department. If additional films might be needed, you may leave the mobile unit in a safe location just *inside* the isolation area and postpone cleaning until the films are processed. When no further exposures are needed, pull the unit into the corridor for cleaning.

Isolation patients in the radiology department

If it is necessary to transport an infectious patient to the radiology department, the first step is to identify the isolation category involved and prepare for the

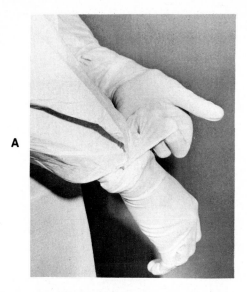

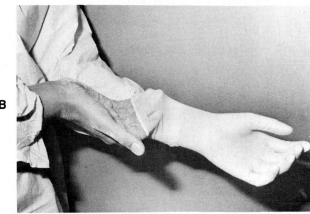

Fig. 5-10. Removing contaminated gloves or those used in isolation rooms. **A,** Grasp first glove from the outside. **B,** Insert your clean fingers *inside* cuff of second glove.

examination accordingly. Cover the stretcher or wheelchair with a sheet, then with another sheet or cotton blanket. Depending on the isolation category involved, you may need to protect yourself and your uniform by wearing a gown, mask, and gloves, if indicated. The patient with respiratory disease should wear a mask while being transported (Fig. 5-12).

Transfer the patient to the wheelchair or stretcher, folding the inner cover around the patient, then the outer cover, and tuck them both in securely. Wash your hands.

When you arrive at the radiology department, take the patient directly into the x-ray room. Protect the table with a sheet. Work with a partner so that one radiographer handles the patient and the other handles the equipment and

Fig. 5-11.

Completion of isolation procedure.

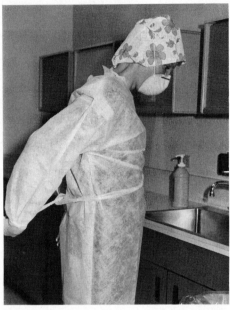

Unfasten waist tie. Loosen gown at neckline. Remove mask and discard.

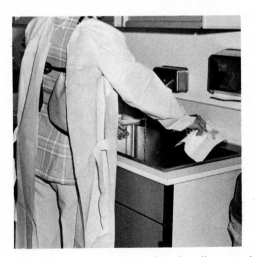

Wash hands, using paper towels to handle controls.

Fig. 5-11.

Completion of isolation procedure—cont'd.

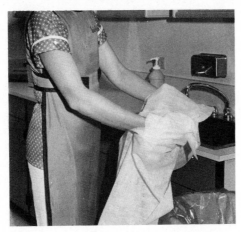

Remove gown, folding contaminated surface inward; discard. *Wash hands* again.

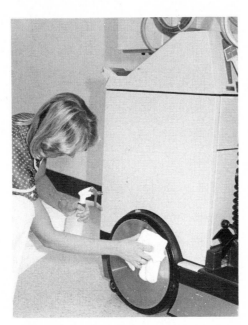

Clean x-ray machine before returning it to the radiology department.

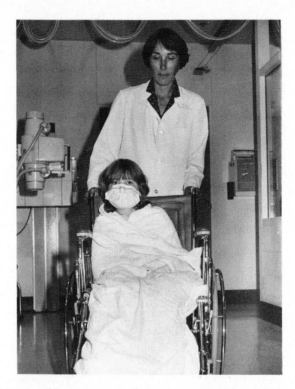

Fig. 5-12. Patient under respiratory isolation is transported to radiology department.

controls, as previously described. Position the patient, and make your exposures as efficiently as possible. Return the patient to the wheelchair or stretcher, re-wrapping the blanket and sheet. Place the sheet from the table and any other contaminated linens in a plastic bag. Place tissues, caps, and other disposable contaminated materials in a paper bag. Put these bags on the wheelchair or stretcher, and return them to the isolation unit for disposal.

On returning the patient to bed, place contaminated linens in the isolation hamper, remove your gloves, wash your hands, and remove your gown as previously described. Clean the wheelchair or stretcher, rewash your hands, and return to the radiology department. During this period, your partner finishes cleaning any other equipment used, including the table, and completes the task with a thorough handwashing.

PRECAUTIONS FOR COMPROMISED PATIENTS

The compromised patient has a very limited immune status and therefore requires special precautions to avoid exposure to potential infection. These patients may have undergone organ transplants and may be taking immunosuppressant medications. Burn patients and neonates at risk may also require these precautions. They are sometimes used for patients receiving chemotherapy that reduces their resistance.

In the recent past these precautions were referred to as reverse isolation or protective isolation. Federal isolation guidelines published in 1983 eliminated the category of protective isolation, largely because the purpose and procedure are the opposite of those of other isolation categories. The same basic principles still apply, however, and the radiographer may find that these terms are still frequently used in the clinical setting.

Precautions for the compromised patient require that the equipment be cleaned before entering the patient's room. Thorough handwashing is required *before* touching the patient, the bed, or articles handled by the patient. Masks, caps, sterile gowns, and gloves may be worn in the same manner used in the operating room, or a modification of surgical technique may be indicated. The modified technique results in a very high degree of medical asepsis without requiring the rigorous protocol of sterile technique. Specific precautions are posted outside the patient's room.

Under the system of protective precautions, the radiographer who positions the patient is the "clean" member of the team. Wearing protective clothing, as indicated, this radiographer avoids contact with cassettes, the x-ray machine, and other potentially contaminated articles. To cover the cassette properly, this radiographer folds back the edges of the sterile cassette cover and holds it open while the second radiographer places the cassette inside. Care must be taken not to contaminate the outside of the cover (Fig. 5-13). The first radiographer touches only the patient, the bed, and "clean" or sterile items, whereas the second radiographer touches only the equipment, as in isolation methods.

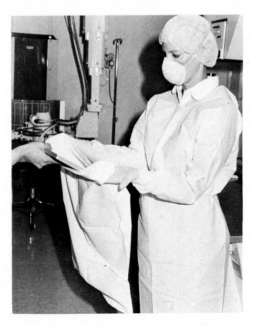

Fig. 5-13. Transfer cassette to sterile cover for protection of patient with compromised resistance.

SURGICAL ASEPSIS

Earlier in this chapter, we defined medical asepsis as a method of reducing the number of pathogenic microorganisms in the environment and intervening in the process by which they are spread. Surgical asepsis, on the other hand, is the complete removal of all organisms and their spores from equipment used to perform patient care or procedures. The linens, gloves, and instruments used in surgery may be the first examples brought to mind, but many other procedures, such as precautions for compromised patients, lumbar puncture, catheterizations, and injections, also require sterile equipment. In addition, some procedures require special skin preparation to prevent pathogens from entering the body. Chapter 9 contains the procedure for performing a skin preparation.

Sterile items used in the radiology department are usually obtained from central supply. Most disposable items, such as small syringes, intravenous sets, and catheterization sets, are sterile when purchased and are protected by a paper or plastic wrap. Reusable items, such as glass syringes and instruments, are wrapped, sterilized, and reissued by central supply.

Sterilization

Although the radiographer is seldom directly involved in the process of sterilization, it is helpful to understand the methods that may be used. Five methods of sterilization are used, some of which are more reliable than others.

Chemical sterilization involves the immersion and soaking of clean objects in a bath of germicidal solution. Sterilization depends on the solution's strength and temperature and the length of time of immersion, all of which are difficult to control accurately. Contamination of the solution or the object being sterilized may occur and is not easily detectable. For this reason, chemical sterilization is one of the less satisfactory methods for providing surgical asepsis and is not recommended. If chemical sterilization must be used, be certain to follow the chemical manufacturer's instructions completely.

Boiling is a method of sterilizing with moist heat that is still used under certain circumstances. A rarely used instrument or a nondisposable item that is needed quickly may be cleaned, completely immersed in water, and boiled for 12 minutes. As with chemical sterilization, this process has no indicator to ensure that the proper conditions for sterilization have been achieved. In addition, several organisms are resistant to this method, making it unacceptable for use in the surgical suite.

Dry heat, such as that in an oven, is used on rare occasions when moist heat is inadvisable. The amount of time needed for sterilization varies from 1 to 6 hours at a temperature range of 329° to 338° F (165° to 170° C).

Items that would be damaged by moist heat are usually sterilized with a mixture of gases (Freon and ethylene oxide) heated to 135° F (57° C). *Gas sterilization* is used primarily for electrical, plastic, and rubber items and for optical ware. Telephones, stethoscopes, blood pressure cuffs, and other equipment used in isolation rooms may be sterilized in this manner.

This treatment sterilizes very effectively but has one drawback: since the gases used are poisonous, they must be dissipated by means of aeration in a

Fig. 5-14.

Establishing a sterile field.

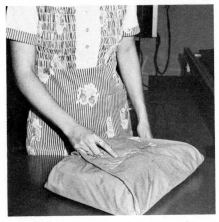

First, check date and sterilization indicator on pack.

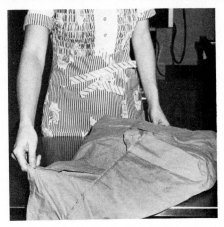

Open first corner away from you.

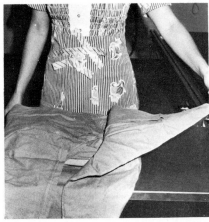

Next, open each side by grasping corner tips.

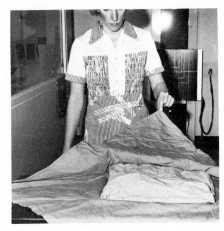

Open remaining corner.

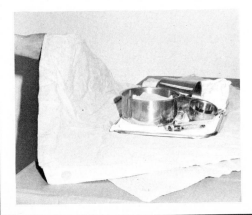

Open inner wrap in the same manner, and sterile field is established.

controlled environment. Aeration is a slow process, and therefore it is important to send items for gas sterilization to central supply well in advance of the time they will be used. A note indicating the date and hour the item is needed will help the staff plan their workload effectively.

Autoclaving, or steam sterilization under pressure, is the quickest and most convenient means of sterilization for items that can withstand heat. Higher temperatures can be achieved under pressure, making this an extremely effective method.

One advantage of steam sterilization is that indicators to ensure sterility have been developed (frequently in the form of tape) that change color when the required conditions have been met. Steam must penetrate to all surfaces of any item to be sterilized. When bulky items are wrapped before autoclaving, an indicator is often placed inside the package as well as outside. Radiographers are responsible for correctly recognizing the sterilization indicators used in their clinical facility.

Preparations must be made before starting a surgical procedure, and the radiographer may be responsible for assembling the needed equipment. Most minor procedures today use disposable equipment, which is wrapped in paper or plastic. Directions on the package are usually clear and precise. The time taken to read them well in advance increases self-confidence when assisting the physician.

Sterile fields

Nondisposable equipment that has been processed by central supply is double-wrapped in cloth or heavy paper and sealed with indicator tape. Such packages are wrapped in a standardized manner and are always opened using the following method. Place the pack on a clean surface within reach of the physician. Just before the procedure begins, break the seal and open the pack. Unfold the first corner away from you, then unfold the two sides. Pull the front fold down toward you and drop it. Do not touch the inner surface. The inner wrap is opened in the same manner. You have now established a sterile field (Fig. 5-14).

Other sterile items wrapped separately may now be added to the sterile field. To do this, grasp the object through the wrapping with one hand. With the other hand, unseal the wrappings, allowing them to fall down over your wrist. Hold the edges of the wrapper with your free hand, and drop the object onto the sterile field without releasing the wrapper (Fig. 5-15). Sponges, gloves, and other small items are often supplied in "peel-down" paper wraps. Following the instructions, separate the paper layers, invert the package, and allow the object to fall onto the sterile field without being contaminated (Fig. 5-16).

It may be necessary to add a liquid medium to the tray. After reading the label three times, position the label toward your hand, remove the cap, pour the first few drops over the bottle's lip into the wastebasket or sink, pour the required amount into the sterile receptacle on the tray, show the physician the label, and recap the bottle. By discarding the first small amount poured, you "wash" the container's lip and avoid the possibility of contaminating the tray (Fig. 5-17).

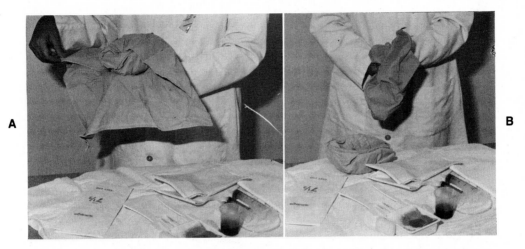

Fig. 5-15. Adding double-wrapped item to sterile field. **A,** Holding item in nondominant hand, open outer wrap; open first fold away from your body. **B,** Avoid contamination by holding corners of wrap while dropping item onto tray.

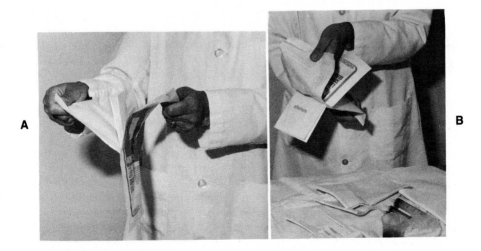

Fig. 5-16. Adding gloves or other items to sterile field from "peel-down" wrap. **A,** Separate wrap as indicated on package. **B,** Invert package, allowing them to drop onto field.

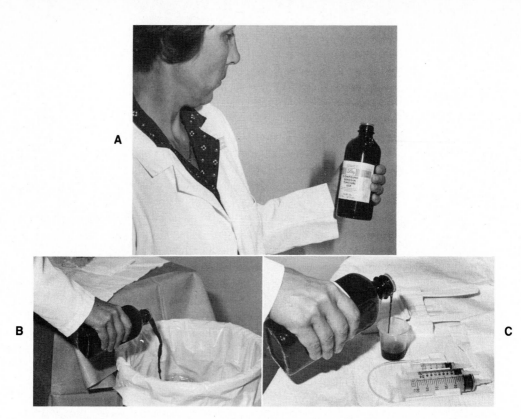

Fig. 5-17. Adding liquid to a sterile field. **A,** Read the label three times. **B,** Flush lip of container by pouring small amount into waste container. **C,** Pour required amount into receptacle on tray, taking care not to contaminate field.

Sterile gowning and gloving

This discussion presumes that the radiographer is preparing a sterile field in which someone else will work and is not the person who will handle the sterile equipment. It is best for the items on the sterile field to be arranged by a person wearing a sterile gown and gloves (Fig. 5-18), that is, one who is "scrubbed in." When a nonscrubbed person must manipulate sterile items, a transfer forceps is used. This long-handled ring forceps may be wrapped separately or found upright in a container of chemical disinfectant. Unwrap or remove the forceps from the container, grasping the handles firmly without touching the remainder of the instrument. Keep the forceps, tip down, above your waist and in your sight at all times. After use, return it to the container or the wrapper with the tips in a sterile field and handles protruding so you can use them again. Do not reach across the sterile field.

If a procedure must be postponed, *do not* open the tray. If it is already open, cover it immediately with a sterile drape or discard it, since airborne contamination is just as serious as a break in sterile technique. For this reason the use of mask and gloves is recommended for even relatively minor procedures.

Following proper procedure, all reusable items must be thoroughly cleaned and returned to central supply. Items must be free of all residue so that the sterilizing agent can penetrate to all surfaces. Thorough cleaning is very important and is most easily accomplished when done promptly.

These standard principles are to be followed regarding surgical asepsis:

1. *Any sterile object or field touched by an unsterile object or person becomes contaminated.* Never reach across a sterile field. Organisms may fall from your arm into the field. Reaching also increases the chance of brushing the area with your uniform.

Fig. 5-18. | **Gloving technique.**

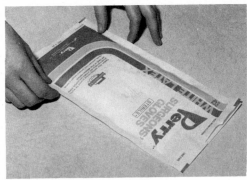
Wash your hands. Obtain gloves and check for correct sizes.

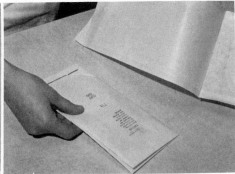
Open outer wrap to expose folded inner wrap.

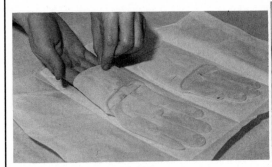
Open inner wrap, touching only outer surface. Expose gloves with open ends facing you.

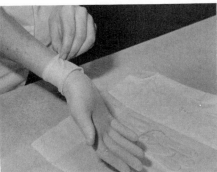
Put on first glove, touching only inner surface of folded cuff.

Fig. 5-18.

Gloving technique—cont'd.

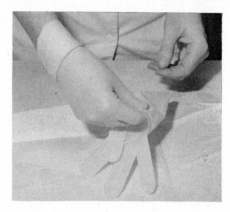

Using gloved hand, grasp second glove *under* cuff.

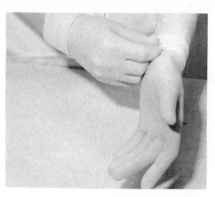

Put on second glove and unfold cuff.

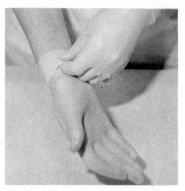

Insert fingers under cuff on first glove and unfold cuff.

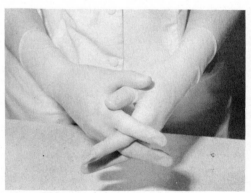

Gloving complete. Keep hands in front of body at safe distance from uniform to avoid contamination.

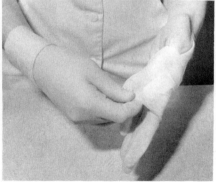

Remove gloves by inverting them as you pull them off.

2. *If you suspect an item is contaminated, discard it.* This includes items that are damp (moisture permits the transfer of bacteria from the outside to the inside of a wrapped set) and items that have the seal broken or on which the indicator tape has not assumed the correct color.
3. *Do not pass between the physician and the sterile field.*
4. *Never leave a sterile area unattended.* If the field is accidentally contaminated (e.g., by a fly or a patient reaching for glasses), no one would know.

We cannot overemphasize the importance of developing a "sterile conscience." This refers to an awareness of sterile technique and the responsibility for telling the person in charge whenever you contaminate a field or observe its contamination by someone else. The inconvenience of reestablishing a sterile field may make a beginning student reluctant to speak out about apparent breaks in technique. Physicians and co-workers may not seem to appreciate your challenge at the moment, but your professionalism and concern for the patient's welfare will be reflected in the confidence that team members place in your aseptic technique.

CONCLUSION

Infection control covers a vast span of possibilities that includes minimizing the spread of the common cold, preventing postoperative infections, and avoiding an exposure to HIV from contaminated blood that could lead to death from AIDS. Radiographers must be aware of both the subtle and the potentially devastating possibilities of infection to themselves and to their patients. Aseptic techniques begin with a commitment to proper practices and are implemented through the conscientious application of knowledge and skill.

Study questions

1. Mr. Mowrey was admitted through the emergency room with a staphylococcal infection caused by leg trauma. List some persons who might become contaminated with his microorganisms if proper isolation technique is not used.
2. Name the type of isolation necessary for Mr. Mowrey, and describe the methods used to implement it.
3. In protective precautions, who wears the mask, the patient or the staff? Why?
4. If a patient with an infectious respiratory condition must be transported to the radiology department, who wears a mask? Why? Is handwashing necessary in this type of isolation?

6

Medications and Their Administration

Objectives

At the conclusion of this chapter, the student will be able to:

1. Define the term *standing order*.
2. Explain what is meant by side effects.
3. Give an example of a trade name and a generic name of a medication typically seen in the radiology department.
4. Demonstrate how to look up a medication in the *Physician's Desk Reference* (PDR).
5. Demonstrate the steps used in the administration of oral medication.
6. List five routes of medication administration.
7. Identify the antecubital vein used for intravenous (IV) injections.
8. Demonstrate the steps taken to discontinue an IV infusion.
9. State the average rate of flow for IV fluids expressed in drops per minute.
10. Identify the sites used for intramuscular injections.

Vocabulary list

1. ampule
2. anesthetic
3. angina pectoris
4. boggy
5. cathartic
6. dehydration
7. edema
8. extravasation
9. generic
10. hematoma
11. hydrostatic pressure
12. infiltration
13. intradermal
14. intramuscular
15. parenteral
16. PDR
17. pledget
18. pulmonary edema
19. radiopaque
20. registered trademark
21. side effects
22. standing orders
23. subcutaneous
24. sublingual
25. synergistic
26. topical
27. vial

THE RADIOGRAPHER'S ROLE

Patients often arrive at the radiology department with intravenous (IV) infusions running and sometimes with a medication pump that delivers measured amounts of drugs. If the pump is set up for self-administration of pain medication, the patient can administer the agent as needed to meet the need for pain relief. Radiographers must monitor these systems while the patients are in their care, but the nursing service is responsible for the initiation of most routine medication administration. Patients who must not miss a dose in their prescribed medical regimen have their medications brought to them by the nurse responsible for their care.

Radiographers become more involved in medication administration when medications are given for specific reasons related to radiographic procedures. Examples include radiopaque drugs injected or ingested to provide radiographic contrast, anesthetic agents injected before the insertion of arterial catheters, and sedation to calm the patient and relieve pain during invasive procedures and magnetic resonance imaging (MRI) examinations. Medications may also be required if a sudden change in a patient's status, such as an allergic reaction, requires emergency medical intervention.

Radiographers may be expected to administer medications or contrast media if state regulations and hospital policies permit this. Otherwise, their role is supportive, with responsibility for preparing the medication, checking the patient identification, reassuring the patient, assisting the physician with administration, and monitoring the patient's progress after the medication has been given.

When medications are given in the radiology department, a physician selects the drug, determines the route of administration, and prescribes the exact dosage. *No medication is ever given without a physician's order.* The order may be either written or verbal and may sometimes be in the form of a standing order. In many states the radiographer is not allowed to accept medication orders by telephone. Verbal orders given in the radiology department should be written or countersigned by the physician before leaving the area. Since this aspect of patient care carries a high potential for medicolegal problems, for your own protection, you must be familiar with the rules governing medication administration in your state as well as in your institution.

The *standing order* is a written policy signed by a physician and applies to patients under specific conditions as stated in the order. For example, many radiology departments have standing orders to administer a cathartic preparation before certain radiographic examinations. In this case a standing order would state which examinations require the preparation, the name and amount of the drug, and any patient conditions that would preclude implementation of the order. It would be signed by the radiologist.

Although the extensive knowledge of drugs expected of a pharmacist or a nurse is not expected of a radiographer, it is very helpful to become familiar with the names, dosages, and routes of administration for those medications frequently used in the radiology department. If this seems intimidating to you, be reassured that only a limited number of drugs and a few standard dosages of those drugs are used with any regularity. Knowledge of these medications greatly facilitates the task of assisting the physician and aids in determining whether departmental stocks of medications and medication supplies are adequate. It also enables the alert radiographer to prevent errors by questioning and double-checking any medication orders or records that seem unusual or inappropriate.

Any drug may produce side effects in certain patients. Radiographers use this knowledge to prepare for untoward drug reactions and to recognize and report signs and symptoms of side effects as they occur. This awareness is very important, since radiographers usually have the most direct contact with patients during their stay in the radiology department and are often the first to observe the onset of medication responses that could have serious consequences. For information on responding to drug reactions, see Chapter 7.

NOMENCLATURE AND PROPERTIES OF MEDICATIONS

Table 6-1 provides a list of common drugs that the radiographer should be familiar with and includes those stocked for emergency use. Note that each medication has a *generic name* that identifies its chemical family. The same generic substance may be manufactured by several different companies and given a different proprietary or *trade name* by each. For example, a synthetic antibacterial containing trimethoprim and sulfamethoxazole is produced by Roche under the name Bactrim and by Burroughs Wellcome as Septra. For some drugs the generic and trade names are used interchangeably. For instance, the generic term epinephrine is used just as frequently as the trade name Adrenalin for this common emergency drug. Since medications may be ordered by either generic or trade names, the radiographer should be familiar with both terms. When the radiologist calls for epinephrine, the knowledgeable radiographer will reach for the Adrenalin without having to read the small print on each container in the emergency drug box.

The study of drugs is an ongoing process, since new medications are constantly being added to the medical repertoire. In addition, no single textbook can provide information for all contingencies. Therefore the radiographer should be acquainted with other methods of obtaining medication facts on a continuing basis. One useful resource is the information sheet enclosed in each drug package. The U.S. Food and Drug Administration (FDA) requires that all drug packages include the following data: trade name, generic name, chemical composition, chemical strength, usual dose, indications, contraindications, and reported side effects. Package inserts from frequently used drugs may be kept on file in the radiology department to avoid the necessity of opening a package when this information is needed. If you collect and study inserts from the drugs used most frequently, you will soon develop a working knowledge and useful base of information about common medications.

Another useful resource is a reference work of medication information, such as the *Physician's Desk Reference* (PDR). This book, which is published annually, lists drugs alphabetically by generic class, trade names, and according to their use. A separate section indexes the products made by each manufacturer. In the product description, you will find information similar to that found in the package inserts. The radiology department library usually includes a PDR, and the radiographer should become familiar with its use.

Table 6-1

Categorized table of some common medications*

Category	Effect	Examples
Adrenergics	Stimulate the sympathetic nervous system, causing constriction of blood vessels, increased cardiac output, rise in blood pressure, and relaxation of smooth muscle lining of the respiratory tract	Epinephrine, (Adrenalin), ephedrine, isoproterenol hydrochloride (Isuprel), metaraminol bitartrate (Aramine), phenylephrine hydrochloride (Neo-Synephrine)
Adrenergic blocking agents	Block the production of epinephrine in the body, thereby causing dilation of blood vessels, decreased cardiac output, and drop in blood pressure; used as antihypertensive agents	Guanethidine sulfate (Ismelin), methyldopa
Analgesics	Relieve pain	Acetaminophen (Tylenol), aspirin, codeine, meperidine (Demerol), methadone, morphine, phenacetin
Anesthetics	Promote loss of feeling or sensation	General: sodium pentothal, halothane (Fluothane), nitrous oxide Local: Xylocaine
Antiarrhythmics (antidysrhythmics)	Prevent or relieve cardiac arrhythmias (dysrhythmias)	Procainamide hydrochloride (Pronestyl), quinidine sulfate, lidocaine (Xylocaine)
Antibacterials	Suppress the growth of bacteria	Internal: penicillins, tetracyclines, sulfadiazine, erythromycin External: sulfonamides, thimerosal (Merthiolate), iodine preparations, hydrogen peroxide, hexachlorophene (pHisoHex)
Anticholinergics	Depress the parasympathetic nervous system and act as antispasmodics of smooth muscle tissue; decrease contractions, saliva, bronchial mucus, digestive secretions, and perspiration; used as preparation for surgery and bronchoscopy to suppress secretions	Atropine, belladonna, propantheline bromide (Pro-Banthine), scopolamine (Hyoscine)

*Generic names of drugs begin with lower-case letters. Trade names are in parentheses and are capitalized.

Continued.

(Table 6-1)

A categorized table of some common medications—cont'd

Category	Effect	Example
Anticoagulants	Inhibit the clotting mechanism of the blood; used to keep IV lines and arterial catheters open during diagnostic procedures	Heparin, warfarin (Coumadin)
Anticonvulsants	Inhibit convulsions	Phenytoin (Dilantin), trimethadione (Tridione)
Antidepressants	Relieve or prevent depression	Amitriptyline hydrochloride (Elavil), imipramine hydrochloride (Tofranil)
Antiemetics	Relieve or prevent vomiting	Trimethobenzamide hydrochloride (Tigan), prochlorperazine (Compazine)
Antifungals	Treat or prevent fungal infections	Systemic: griseofulvin Topical: Tinactin
Antihistamines	Relieve the symptoms of allergic reactions	Diphenhydramine hydrochloride (Benadryl), pheniramine maleate (Trimeton), chlorpheniramine maleate (Chlor-Trimeton)
Antiperistaltics	Slow peristalsis of the gastrointestinal tract	Tincture of opium (paregoric) (Lomotil)
Antipyretics	Reduce fever	Aspirin, acetaminophen (Tylenol)
Antitussives	Prevent coughing	Codeine, dextromethorphan hydrobromide (Romilar)
Barbiturates	Depress the central nervous system (CNS), respirations, and blood pressure and induce sleep	Pentobarbital sodium (Nembutal), secobarbital sodium (Seconal), phenobarbital
Cardiac depressants	Restrain or slow the heart's activity	Quinidine, procainamide hydrochloride (Pronestyl)
Cardiac stimulants	Strengthen and tone the heart, increasing cardiac output	Digitalis, gitalin (Gitaligin), lanatoside C (Cedilanid)
Cathartics	Promote defecation	Bisacodyl (Dulcolax), castor oil, magnesium sulfate
Contrast media; see Chapter 9		
Diuretics	Stimulate the flow of urine	Chlorothiazide (Diuril), furosemide (Lasix), acetazolamide (Diamox)
Emetics	Induce vomiting	Ipecac
Hypoglycemics	Lower the blood sugar level	Insulin, chlorpropamide (Diabinese), tolbutamide (Orinase)

Table 6-1

A categorized table of some common medications—cont'd

Category	Effect	Example
Narcotics	Analgesics/sedatives with a potential for addiction; classified as controlled substances under the Harrison Act	Morphine, meperidine (Demerol), codeine
Narcotic antagonists	Prevent or counteract respiratory depression and other depressive effects of morphine and related drugs	Nalorphine hydrochloride (Nalline), levallorphan tartrate (Lorfan)
Radioactive isotopes	Radioactive forms of elements used for diagnostic and treatment	Iodine-131, cobalt-60
Sedatives	Depress and relax the CNS and reduce mental activity	Barbiturates, paraldehyde, chloral hydrate
Skeletal muscle relaxants	Relax skeletal or striated muscle tissue	Carisoprodol (Soma), succinylcholine chloride (Anectine Chloride), tubocurarine
Stimulants	Stimulate the CNS	Caffeine and sodium benzoate, amphetamines (Benzedrine, Dexedrine), theobromine, theophylline
	Stimulate the respiratory system	Nikethamide (Coramine), caffeine and sodium benzoate, doxapram (Dopram)
Tranquilizers	Reduce anxiety	Minor: hydroxyzine pamoate (Vistaril), diazepam (Valium), chlordiazepoxide hydrochloride (Librium), meprobamate (Miltown)
		Major: chlorpromazine hydrochloride (Thorazine), thioridazine (Mellaril), trifluoperazine (Stelazine)
Vasodilators	Relax the walls of blood vessels, permitting a greater flow of blood	Isosorbide dinitrate (Sorbitrate), Trinitroglycerol, hydralazine hydrochloride (Apresoline)

Knowledge of some common medications helps you evaluate changes in the condition of patients in your care. Reference to the medication record in the patient's chart may help you determine whether a change in status is caused by medication or a deterioration in the patient's condition. For example, anticholinergics such as atropine cause a dry mouth. Narcotics may slow the respiratory rate, and vasodilators may cause the blood pressure to drop. Such effects are the usual consequence of the specific medication and are taken into account when the drug is prescribed.

Untoward or adverse side effects, on the other hand, may range from mild nausea, flushing, or diarrhea to cardiac arrest or other life-threatening states. Hives, respiratory distress, or abrupt changes in blood pressures are all symptoms demanding a physician's immediate intervention. (See Chapter 7 for further details on response to allergic reactions.) Since many drugs have a synergistic effect when taken together, the physician must have the patient's chart available when a new medication is ordered.

FREQUENTLY USED MEDICATIONS

The following medications are used regularly in many radiology and special imaging departments. These general descriptions illustrate how such medications are used but are not meant to be exclusive. The specific drugs used at your institution may be different while meeting the same needs.

Antiallergic medications

Diphenhydramine (Benadryl) is the most frequently used antihistamine. It also has sedative and anticholinergic (drying) side effects. It can be given orally in advance to patients who might be expected to have an allergic reaction. For adults, the usual oral dose is 25 to 50 mg, and for children weighing more than 20 pounds, the dosage is 12.5 to 25 mg. Benadryl may also be given intramuscularly (IM) or intravenously (IV) if the patient has allergic reaction. The dosage is 10 to 50 mg IV or IM, up to 100 mg as necessary. The maximum safe dosage in a 24-hour period is 400 mg.

For patients with an acute allergic reaction, epinephrine (Adrenalin) is administered subcutaneously (SC), IM, or IV. To control angioedema, shock, or respiratory distress, the physician administers a small dose (0.2 to 1 ml of 1:1000 solution) and increases the dosage if required.

When patients with a severe or incapacitating allergic response do not appear to respond to the treatment just described, methylprednisolone (Solu-Medrol) may be administered IV. This is a corticosteroid that acts as an antiinflammatory agent, preventing or reducing *edema* (swelling) of the tracheobronchial tree. This treatment minimizes the possibility of respiratory arrest. Solu-Medrol is provided in a special two-compartment vial with the diluting fluid and soluble powder separated by a plunger/stopper. The directions for mixing are provided, but you should become familiar with the preparation of this and all these common medications *before* the need arises.

Analgesics and narcotics

These medications are called *controlled substances*. These drugs have a high potential for abuse and misuse and therefore are kept in a locked container. They must be counted and listed on forms that give the date, patient's name, dose, and name and title of the person administering the medication. Use of these drugs is monitored by the U.S. Drug Enforcement Administration (DEA).

Pain medications (analgesics) are given not only to help the patient cope with painful procedures but also to lessen possible pain originating before the procedure that makes it difficult for the patient to cooperate. Although the pain might be the reason for the examination, it might also be a chronic problem that causes enough discomfort to prevent compliance with the examination. For example, a patient may have painful arthritis of the cervical spine that makes it extremely difficult to lie still for the 30 minutes required for MRI of the brain.

Drugs that relieve severe pain are also narcotics, meaning that they induce sleep. Narcotics act by depressing the central nervous system (CNS), relieving pain and producing drowsiness. Excessive doses, however, can result in coma and possible death.

Among the most frequently used narcotics are morphine (morphine sulfate, typically referred to as MS) and meperidine (Demerol). These injectable medications are given in a dosage of 50 to 100 mg (Demerol) or 10 to 30 mg (morphine). Fentanyl (Sublimaze), another narcotic analgesic, is given to patients who are sensitive to other narcotics or who are not responding to such medications with adequate pain relief. The physician determines the dosage of this highly potent medication based on age, weight, use of other drugs, and the procedure involved. The action of Sublimaze is almost immediate and lasts 30 to 60 minutes after IV administration. It is supplied in a strength of 50 micrograms per milliliter (μg/ml), and the usual dose is 1 to 2 ml. Respiratory depression peaks 5 to 10 minutes after injection and may last for several hours, depending on the dosage.

Patients who have received *any* CNS depressant must be monitored closely. Respiratory depression is a life-threatening side effect. A narcotic antagonist and resuscitation equipment should be immediately available. Since patients may be some distance from the radiographer during computed tomography (CT) or MRI, a pulse oximeter is attached to the patient's finger or toe. A digital readout of the pulse and oxygen saturation of the blood is viewed from the control room. If the oxygen saturation drops to less than 90%, the patient is asked to respond and take a few deep breaths, then is observed closely. If the oxygen saturation continues to drop or the patient does not respond adequately, a physician is notified immediately.

Sedatives and tranquilizers

Sedatives are medications that exert a quieting effect, often inducing sleep. They do not relieve pain as such but may provide relief from muscle tension. Tranquilizers more effectively reduce anxiety and mental tension and often provide some sedation. At low doses, tranquilizers do not impair mental acuity, but as the dosage increases, patients tend to feel drowsy and speech may become slow and slurred. Some patients experience a brief loss of inhibition, similar to alcohol's effect, which causes them to talk and act inappropriately. Individuals taking tranquilizers may have slowed reaction time and thus should not drive or operate machinery.

Phenobarbital and other barbiturates were formerly used as sedatives and preoperative medications. These have been largely supplanted by diazepam. Phenobarbital is still used with other medications to treat patients with seizures.

Diazepam (Valium) and midazolam (Versed) have a tranquilizing effect and may be given with morphine to highly anxious and uncomfortable patients. The dosage of Valium for premedication ranges from 2 to 20 mg given IM or IV. The physician may administer larger doses as needed to achieve relaxation, and very large doses are sometimes given to control a seizure. When injecting Valium IV, give it slowly, taking at least 1 minute for each 5 mg (1 ml) given. Avoid using small veins of the hand and wrist, since Valium is irritating to blood vessels and can possibly cause phlebitis and damage to the vein. *Extravasation,* or infiltration of Valium into surrounding tissues, can be painful, causing irritation and swelling.

Versed is sometimes added to a previous administration of a narcotic or Valium when the desired state of pain relief and relaxation has not been achieved. The initial dose of Versed in this instance is 1 mg and can be increased to a usual maximum of 10 mg at the physician's discretion.

Antagonists

Naloxone (Narcan) counteracts the effects of opiates such as morphine and prevents or reverses respiratory depression, sedation, and hypotension. A rapid reversal of narcotic depression can result in nausea, vomiting, tachycardia, and nervousness. Although Narcan can be administered SC or IM, the most rapid onset of action is obtained with a dilution of Narcan in saline or 5% dextrose and water administered IV. To reverse respiratory depression, 0.1 to 0.2 mg Narcan should be administered IV at 2- to 3-minute intervals until adequate ventilation is achieved.

Flumazenil (Mazicon) is a medication developed to counteract the effect of benzodiazepines such as Valium. Mazicon can antagonize the sedation and the impairment of recall and psychomotor function produced by benzodiazepines. Patients who receive Mazicon should be monitored for resedation, respiratory depression, or other residual effects for up to 2 hours based on the dosage and duration of the benzodiazepine used. For the reversal of conscious sedation by benzodiazepines, the recommended initial dose of Mazicon is 0.2 mg (2 ml) administered IV over 15 seconds. If the desired level of consciousness is not obtained after waiting an additional 45 seconds, additional doses may be given until the desired effect is achieved to a maximum of 1 mg (10 ml). To minimize the possibility of pain or inflammation, Mazicon should be administered through a freely flowing IV line into a large vein. The use of Mazicon has been associated with seizures in patients who have been taking benzodiazepines for long-term sedation.

Local anesthetics

Lidocaine (Xylocaine) is a local anesthetic used to eliminate pain in a specific area before beginning a painful procedure. You may have received such an injection before having dental work or when having stitches placed to close a wound. Xylocaine is provided in a variety of strengths and is available both with or without epinephrine. The addition of epinephrine causes constriction of adjacent blood vessels and localizes the anesthetic effect to the immediate area. If your department stocks more than one type, be sure you understand clearly which one the physician requires.

Succinylcholine chloride

When working in a trauma unit or emergency department, the radiographer may occasionally come in contact with patients who have received succinylcholine chloride (commonly referred to as "succs"). This skeletal muscle relaxant is sometimes given to facilitate insertion of an endotracheal airway or to initiate diagnostic studies and treatment for patients who are combative because of shock, fear, or intoxication. Since all muscles are temporarily paralyzed, artificial respiration is given, and patients are monitored closely until the effects of the medication wear off. Succinylcholine does not cause the patient to become unconscious, and since the period of paralysis is very short, these patients are frequently agitated or combative as the paralysis dissipates.

• • •

Some of the drugs just discussed can cause respiratory depression and *any* of them could cause an allergic reaction in a sensitized individual. Know where the resuscitation equipment and oxygen are kept, and be familiar with the code routine of your institution (see Chapter 7).

This discussion has touched on some of the frequently used medications of importance to radiographers. Wherever you work, you must become thoroughly familiar with the protocols of your institution. Your card file with the package inserts serves as a handy tool to help you stay current in your knowledge of these drugs' dosage, actions, and side effects.

MEDICATION ADMINISTRATION

The information in this section provides a basis for assisting the physician in medication administration but is not intended as a substitute for directions from the physician. Supervised clinical practice and familiarity with institutional procedures are required to implement this knowledge. A practical memory device can serve to protect both the patient and the radiographer when medications must be administered. This is called the *five rights* system:

1. The right dose
2. Of the right medication
3. To the right patient
4. At the right time
5. By the right route

Dosage

The metric system, with which you are already familiar, is usually used for measuring medications. Liquids are measured in units from liters (L, slightly more than a quart) down to milliliters (ml), which are thousandths of a liter. One milliliter is equal to 1 cubic centimeter (cc), and 1 ounce equals 30 ml. Since liquid agents are often diluted for use, the strength is expressed as a ratio of the amount of the drug to the total volume of solution. For example, 1:1000 indicates a dilution of one part drug to 1000 parts of water or other solvent.

If the active ingredient is a solid, it is measured by weight in grams (g), milligrams (mg), or micrograms (μg). The strength of solids dissolved in a liquid is designated in terms of weight per volume, often mg/ml. You will often need to determine how much liquid will provide a given dose of a solid:

$$\frac{Dose}{Strength} = Volume$$

Example: if the drug is supplied in a strength of 4 mg/ml, and you want to administer 10 mg, you will need 2.5 ml:

$$\frac{10\ mg}{4\ mg/ml} = 2.5\ ml$$

Conversely, you may need to know how much of a solid is delivered in a given volume of liquid:

$$Strength \times Volume = Dose$$

Example: if 2 ml of solution is given and the strength is 4 mg/ml, the dose would be 8 mg:

$$4\ mg/ml \times 2\ ml = 8\ mg$$

Practice these calculations so that you can do them quickly without error whenever you are required to prepare a parenteral medication.

Topical route

The topical route of administration can be used when a drug is applied to a limited area for a local effect, such as the calamine lotion used to relieve the itch of poison ivy. Other topical medications are used for a systemic effect. One topical drug is frequently used by patients with heart conditions. When coronary arteries are unable to supply the heart muscle with sufficient nutrients and oxygen, a crushing pain results. This is called *angina pectoris.* When nitroglycerin is administered *sublingually,* or beneath the tongue, it is absorbed directly into the bloodstream, dilating the coronary arteries. This helps relieve the pain by improving circulation to the heart muscle. Patients with "angina" should have their medication with them during x-ray procedures. An emergency supply of nitroglycerin is usually stocked in the radiology department.

Other topical medications are applied through the skin in "paste" form or on small adhesive disks. These include a medication to prevent vertigo (Antivert or scopolamine) and a medication to increase vascular dilation (nifedipine).

Oral route

The oral route is easiest and most familiar. Oral medications are supplied in a variety of forms, including tablets, capsules, granules, and liquids. Tablets and capsules are swallowed with varying amounts of liquid, usually water. Liquid medications are usually taken with water as well. Granules are mixed with a specified amount of liquid. Follow the directions on the package insert.

One way to minimize errors in the administration of drugs is to establish a set routine and follow it unfailingly. The following steps serve as a guide to establishing a procedure for the administration of oral medications.

⇒ Administering oral medications

1. Wash your hands.
2. Obtain the proper medication, and read the label.
3. Prepare the medication tray with a medicine cup and a glass of water (if appropriate). Read the label again.
4. Show the physician the label, and pour the correct amount of medication directly into the medicine cup. When pouring liquids, hold the label against the palm of your hand so that it will stay clean and legible.
5. If requested by the physician to administer the medication, check the patient's identification, stay with the patient while the medication is swallowed, and offer water if permitted.
6. Return the tray, and discard the used water and medicine cup.
7. Wash your hands again.
8. Chart the medication.

Parenteral route

While patients may prefer to take medications orally, some drugs cause irritation of the gastrointestinal tract, cannot be absorbed by this route, or must be given by a route that will produce a very rapid response. By using the parenteral route, medications can be injected directly into the body. Parenteral injections may be of several types and are classified according to the depth of the injection.

Intravenous administration is the parenteral route that offers the most immediate results in terms of effect. This extremely important route is covered in detail later in this chapter.

Subcutaneous (under the skin) medications are injected at a 45-degree angle using a ⅝-inch needle with a size 23 to 25 gauge. Syringes used for subcutaneous injections are usually 2 ml or smaller in size, since it is painful to inject a large quantity beneath the skin. The most convenient areas for subcutaneous injections are on the upper arm and on the outer aspect of the thigh.

Intramuscular (into the muscle) injections are sometimes given in larger amounts. The syringe may be larger (up to 5 ml) and the needle size is also larger, usually 22 gauge. The injection is given into the deltoid muscle of the upper arm, the upper outer quadrant of the gluteus maximus muscle in the hip, or the vastus lateralis muscle of the lateral thigh (Fig. 6-1). For children under 5 years of age, the vastus lateralis site is preferred to the gluteus site. Since the gluteus maximus muscle only develops fully through walking and running, a danger of damage to the sciatic nerve exists when injections are given into this area before the muscle is sufficiently developed. Injections are not usually given into the anterior thigh because this site is extremely painful and the discomfort may persist for several days.

Intradermal injections (between the layers of the skin) were formerly given to test the sensitivity of patients to contrast media. Experience over the years has proved that a complete history is a more accurate predictor of allergic reactions than the intradermal "skin test." Thus the radiographer is not likely to encounter this procedure. A tuberculin syringe is frequently used for intradermal injections, since it is finely calibrated and comes with a very small (26- gauge) needle. The anterior surface of the forearm is a typical site for these injections.

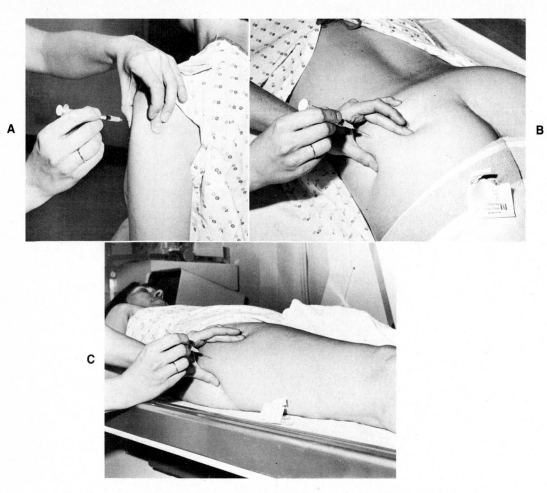

Fig. 6-1. Intramuscular injection sites. **A,** Deltoid muscle. **B,** Gluteus maximus muscle. **C,** Vastus lateralis muscle.

Preparation for injection.   To prepare for any parenteral injection, the radiographer must assemble the proper syringe and needle and an alcohol pledget for cleansing the skin. Next, the medication is obtained, and the label is read carefully. This is essential to be absolutely certain that it is the correct drug and the proper strength. The label indicates not only the name of the medication and the amount per ml, but also gives an expiration date, past which the drug should not be used. When medications are not used frequently (as in an emergency kit or on a crash cart), they should be checked often and out-of-date supplies discarded and replaced. Never borrow medication or equipment from the crash cart. If supplies have been used for an emergency, they should be replaced as soon as possible.

If a drug is supplied in ampule form, a small file is needed to nick the neck of the ampule. The top then snaps off easily. Use a 2×2 inch gauze sponge to protect your fingers when opening the ampule, since the glass may break unevenly and cut your hand (Fig. 6-2). Next, attach the needle to the syringe securely, and remove the needle cover, taking care not to contaminate the needle. Withdraw the required amount of the medication into the syringe, and hold the syringe to the light to check for air bubbles. If bubbles appear, hold the syringe with the needle pointing up, and tap the side of the syringe. As the bubbles rise, they can be ejected with gentle pressure on the plunger. The removal of air is essential to accurate dosage measurement and may also affect patient safety. Now, read the label again. The ampule is retained until after the drug has been administered and charted. Before the drug is administered, the radiographer shows the physician the ampule and the syringe while stating aloud what has been done. After administration, the medication is charted and the ampule, together with any remaining medication, is discarded.

If the medication is supplied in a vial, several variations exist in the preparation procedure. First, pull off the protective cap, taking care not to contaminate the underlying surface. Vials have rubber stoppers through which a needle can be inserted. Since this is a closed system, you must inject a volume of air equal to the amount of fluid you wish to remove. Remove the needle cover, and pull down the plunger of the syringe to the desired reading. Insert the needle through the stopper, and inject the air into the bottle. Invert the bottle, and make sure the needle tip is below the fluid level. Then, pull down the plunger to the desired reading, and check for bubbles. If there are any, dislodge them,

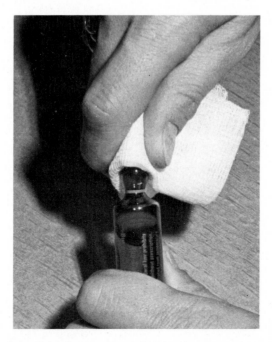

Fig. 6-2. Take time to protect hands when opening ampule.

and inject them into the vial. Withdraw the plunger again until the dosage is correct. Then, remove the needle, replace the needle cover, and proceed as previously described (Fig. 6-3).

The vial was originally designed as a multiple-dose container, but the frequency of contamination is so great that its multiple-use capability is now restricted to use for the same patient on the same day. Vials of local anesthetic are sometimes used repeatedly for the same patient during a radiographic procedure. When using a vial *after* the first time, clean the stopper with an alcohol

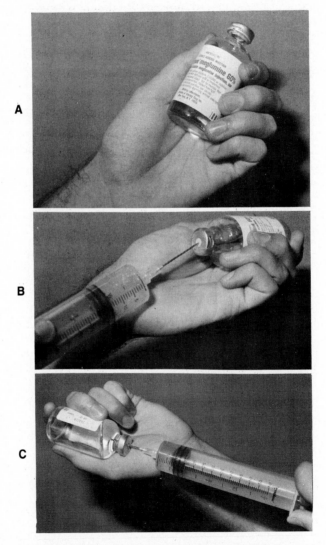

Fig. 6-3. Loading syringe from vial. **A,** Read label carefully. Check for drug name, correct strength, and expiration date. **B,** Pull back on plunger to reading of desired dose. With vial tipped upward, inject air into air space in vial. **C,** Tip vial downward to withdraw solution.

pledget. (Alcohol is not used for the first injection because the stopper is sterile on opening the vial, and alcohol may, in rare instances, produce a toxic effect if accidentally mixed with the medication.) When the procedure is completed, discard the vial and any remaining medication. Some vials are not meant for multiple use and are so marked. Vials have largely been replaced by preloaded syringes that are discarded after use.

Intravenous access

IV fluids and medications are administered to meet specific needs. This route of drug administration allows patients to respond rapidly to medication. The IV injection is used for delivering most emergency medications when an immediate response is critical.

Dehydrated patients may need fluid and electrolyte replacement. The most common replacement fluids are normal saline or a 5% solution of dextrose in water. These solutions are usually stocked in radiology departments. If you are starting or replacing IV fluids, be certain that the solution is correct. Less common solutions or those containing medication may need to be replaced by the nursing service.

The IV route may serve to transport parenteral nutrition or chemotherapy. This is also the route used to inject contrast media in radiographic examinations of the urinary tract and in some CT studies and to provide sedation during invasive procedures and MRI examinations.

IV equipment.   Venipuncture may be accomplished with a hypodermic needle, a butterfly set, or an IV catheter.

The use of hypodermic needles is generally restricted to phlebotomy for obtaining laboratory samples and for single, small injections. Hypodermic needles are supplied in various diameters and lengths. The *gauge* of a needle indicates the diameter, and the gauge increases as the diameter of the bore decreases. An 18-gauge needle is larger around than a 22-gauge needle and delivers a given volume of fluid more rapidly. A 22-gauge needle can be used for much smaller veins; since it makes a smaller hole, excessive bleeding or hematoma is less likely when it is removed. The length of hypodermic needles is measured in inches and may vary from ½ inch, used for accessing IV line ports and for intradermal use, to 4½ inches, used for intrathecal (spinal canal) injections. A 2½-inch length is typical for IV needles, and the usual gauge ranges from 18 to 22 for adults.

A butterfly set is preferable to a conventional hypodermic needle for most IV injections and is often used for direct injections with a syringe. This apparatus consists of a needle with plastic projections on either side that aid in holding the needle during venipuncture and that may be taped to the patient's skin after the needle is in place (Fig. 6-4). This prevents movement of the needle in the vein. Attached to the needle is a short length of tubing with a hub that attaches to a syringe. The syringe is filled from a vial or ampule, and the syringe is then attached to the tubing. Before the butterfly needle is inserted into the vein, the tubing is filled with liquid from the syringe to avoid injecting air into the vein.

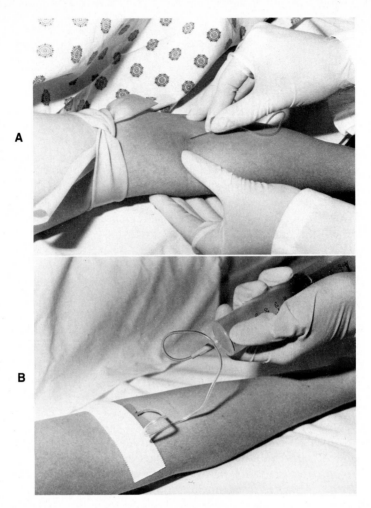

Fig. 6-4. Butterfly set facilitates direct IV injection. **A,** Needle projections provide grip for venipuncture. **B,** Tubing adds stability during injection.

IV catheters are frequently used instead of needles or butterfly sets when repeated or continuous IV injections or infusions will be administered. The IV catheter is a two-part system consisting of a needle that fits inside a flexible plastic catheter. The catheter's hub has wing-shaped plastic projections similar to the butterfly set. The needle portion is not hollow and serves as a stylet to prevent blood flow through the catheter. This combination unit is inserted into the vein, and the catheter is advanced by slipping it forward over the needle. The catheter is then secured with tape, the needle is withdrawn, and the catheter is connected to the supply system. IV fluid, medication, or contrast can now be administered by syringe through an injection port or IV tubing from a hanging bottle or bag.

An intermittent injection port (sometimes called a heparin lock) is a small adapter with a diaphragm that is attached to an IV catheter when more than one injection is anticipated.

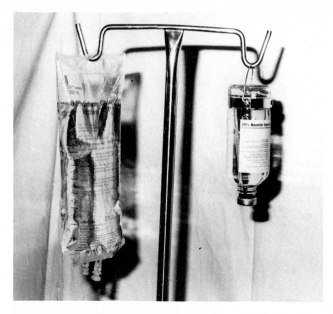

Fig. 6-5. IV fluids are packaged in bottles and in plastic bags.

When a procedure requires the IV infusion of a large volume of fluid, an IV pole and infusion set are needed. Setting up fluid administration equipment is not complicated but is another skill that improves with practice. IV solutions are provided in bottles and plastic bags (Fig. 6-5). The bags have a cap over the sterile port through which the drip chamber of the IV tubing is inserted. The drip chamber is removed from its wrappings and inserted into the sterile port. Care must be taken not to contaminate either component, or both must be discarded.

Solutions supplied in bottles have a removable cap and sometimes a rubber diaphragm covering a rubber stopper. The cap is removed, and the diaphragm is pulled off without touching the stopper. The drip chamber is inserted through the stopper; one must ensure that the clamp on the IV tubing is closed. Now, the bottle or bag may be inverted and hung on the IV pole. After it is in place, the cover at the other end of the IV tubing is removed, the clamp is opened, and the fluid is allowed to run into a basin until the tubing is free of bubbles. The clamp is then closed and the tip covered to keep it sterile. The procedure is illustrated in Fig. 6-6.

Starting an IV line.   The veins most often used for initiating IV lines are found in the anterior forearm, the posterior hand, the radial aspect of the wrist, and the antecubital space (Fig. 6-7). Usually the two antecubital veins on each arm are large enough and near enough to the surface to be easily seen. Although they may be the easiest to locate and to puncture, there are drawbacks to their use. Easy access to these veins is important for emergencies and for routine blood draws. However, overuse may cause these veins to become scarred or

Fig. 6-6.

IV infusion setup.

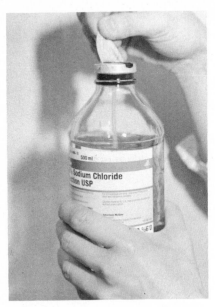

After removing cap, remove diaphragm carefully to avoid contamination.

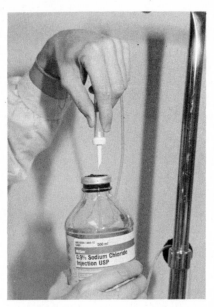

With tubing clamped off, insert drip chamber firmly into access port.

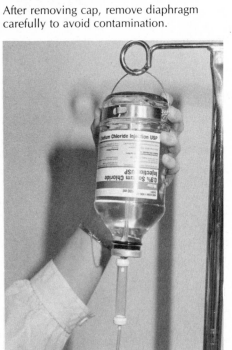

Invert bottle or bag and suspend from pole.

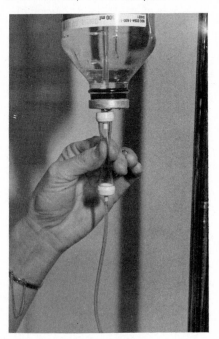

Pinch drip chamber to draw fluid into chamber. Fill chamber about half full.

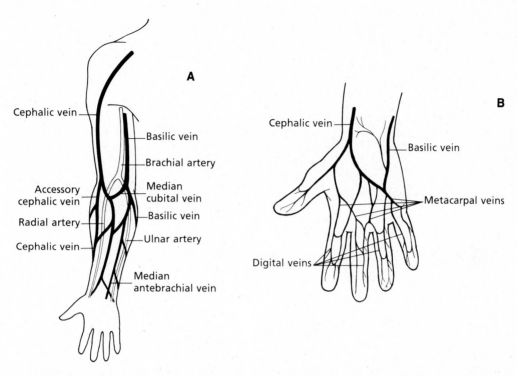

Fig. 6-7. Veins typically used for venipuncture. **A,** Veins of anterior aspect of forearm. **B,** Superficial veins of dorsal aspect of hand.

sclerotic, which can be a serious problem with patients receiving long-term care. When antecubital IV lines remain in place for some time, they may become uncomfortable and inhibit the patient's ability to flex the elbow. Flexion at the elbow may crimp the catheter, preventing IV flow.

For these reasons the nursing service tends to use antecubital veins as a last resort. In imaging departments, however, the IV line is usually placed only for the duration of the procedure, and the use of antecubital veins is acceptable when necessary. A vein of adequate size is essential when a bolus of contrast will be delivered at a rapid rate. For small children, this usually requires an antecubital site.

When placing an IV line in an antecubital vein, a flexible IV catheter should be used. *Never leave a needle in an antecubital vein unless the elbow is restrained in extension by attaching it to an armboard.* Flexion of the elbow with a needle in an antecubital vein ruptures the vein, causing extravasation and hematoma.

To select a vein, first secure the tourniquet around the arm above the elbow.

Fig. 6-8. **Venipuncture using IV catheter.**

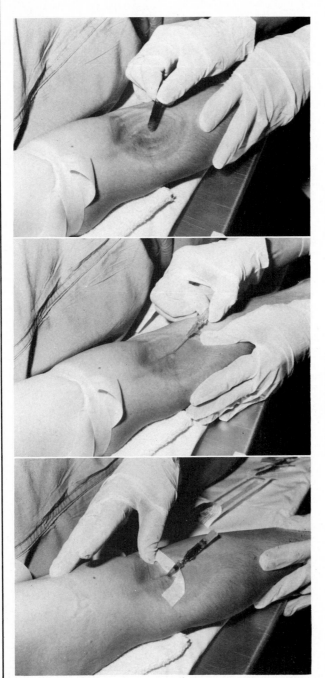

After securing tourniquet and selecting vein, cleanse skin according to protocol for your institution.

Wearing gloves, hold catheter at an acute angle to skin and insert into vein. Advance catheter over needle until hub is against skin. Blood return into catheter and needle hub indicates successful placement.

Secure hub in place with tape.

Fig. 6-8.

Venipuncture using IV catheter—cont'd.

If IV line will remain in place after procedure, treat site with antiseptic ointment and cover with protective film. Add a label with date, time, catheter gauge, and your initials.

Holding pressure on vein near tip of catheter, remove stylet and connect to delivery system. In this illustration, intermittent injection port with attached flush syringe is secured to catheter.

If intermittent injection port is used, flush catheter and discard syringe.

Instruct the patient to open and close the hand a few times and then hold a tight fist. These measures restrict circulation and enlarge the veins, making them easier to identify and to penetrate accurately. The ideal vein can be readily seen and palpated. It is at least twice the diameter of the needle or catheter you plan to use, and the vein appears not to bend or curve for a distance at least equal to the length of the needle or catheter. If a suitable vein is not immediately apparent, let the arm hang down for a few seconds, then gently slap the skin over the area where the vein should appear. This may increase the likelihood that the vein will stand out well. If a suitable vein is still not apparent, remove the tourniquet and begin again with the other arm. Fig. 6-8 shows the step-by-step procedure for initiating an IV line using an IV catheter.

As you practice with classmates, suitable veins may appear readily. In the clinical setting, however, it is sometimes more difficult. Obese patients may have veins that are too deep to be seen or palpated. Elderly patients may have veins that are easily seen but that may roll under the skin or be too crooked to be suitable. For patients who have undergone mastectomy, you must select a vein on the extremity opposite the side of the mastectomy site. Patients who have had extensive IV therapy, especially chemotherapy, may have scarred and sclerotic veins that preclude a routine approach. Infants and children also present challenges. Their small veins may be more difficult to see and feel, and the situation is often complicated by the child's refusal or inability to cooperate. Attempt venipuncture *only* when you have a reasonable expectation of success.

The range of situations in which you feel competent will increase considerably with experience. If a particular patient's situation is beyond your skill level, or if you have attempted venipuncture twice on a patient unsuccessfully, consult another team member. Most hospitals have an IV therapy department with specially trained and highly experienced nurses who will assist you with difficult situations. Some hospital policies state that all IV lines for chemotherapy patients and children under a certain age must be started by IV therapy personnel.

IV medication administration.   When the IV line has been established, IV medications are typically administered through an intermittent injection port or through access ports on IV infusion tubing. After the patient identification and the medication label are checked, the correct dosage is drawn up into a syringe. The access port is then cleansed with alcohol, and the medication is injected through the port. When an intermittent injection port is used, a small amount of flush solution is injected through the port to prevent blood from coagulating inside the catheter. The system is flushed immediately after it is established, and again after each use, with saline or heparin solution. In many institutions, heparin is used as a flush only with a physician's order.

The hazards posed by needle sticks have prompted the development of "needleless" systems such as the Baxter InterLink IV access system (Fig. 6-9). This system facilitates blood draws and IV medication administration without the use of needles. An important feature of the system is a self-healing rubber substance that is used for medication vial caps, intermittent injection ports, and access ports on IV tubing. These caps and ports can be repeatedly penetrated

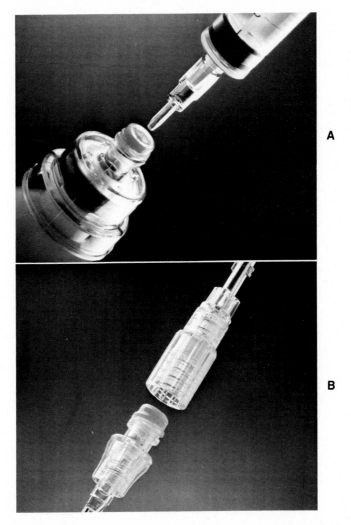

Fig. 6-9. Example of needleless IV access system. **A,** Needle-free safety is facilitated with Baxter InterLink System Vial Adapter, shown here fitted to top of multiple-dose vial. The special adapter, which fits any standard 20 mm neck vial, equips it to accept blunt InterLink Cannula. **B,** When added security is desired, InterLink Threaded Luer Lok Cannula securely connects to InterLink Injection Site without taping. This Luer locking feature provides a secure, sterile, and leak-free connection between IV devices that minimizes contamination through touch. *(Courtesy Baxter Healthcare Corp.)*

by blunt plastic cannulas without damaging their integrity. The blunt cannulas are used to draw up medications and to access established IV lines for blood draws and medication administration. The use of a needleless system greatly reduces the incidence of needle use and its attendant hazards in the health care setting.

Extravasation.   Occasionally IV fluid or medication may accidentally be injected into the tissues surrounding the vein. This extravasation may be both painful and dangerous. The patient is likely to complain of discomfort, and you may observe swelling at the site. The following precautions are employed to minimize the possibility of extravasation: (1) checking for backflow to determine that the catheter or needle is properly situated before injection, (2) immobilizing the needle or catheter at the injection site, and (3) stopping the injection immediately if the patient complains of discomfort at the injection site or if any resistance to injection is felt.

When extravasation does occur, it is necessary to remove the needle and attend to this problem before proceeding with an injection at another site. Assure the patient that the pain is only temporary. Maintain pressure on the vein until bleeding has stopped completely. This will avoid the additional complication of a *hematoma* at the site of the extravasation. After the bleeding has stopped, the application of hot packs or moist heat to the affected area will help alleviate the pain. If hot packs are not readily available, a terry towel may be soaked in water as hot as the hands can tolerate. The towel is then wrung out and wrapped around the arm at the injection site. A dry towel may be wrapped around the wet one to hold in the heat. The hot towel must be replaced with another as soon as it begins to cool and the process repeated until the burning sensation at the injection site is alleviated. It is recommended that an incident report be completed for any extravasation involving a potentially irritating medication or contrast medium. Outpatients should be advised to consult their physicians or to report to the emergency department if inflammation or discomfort persists.

Discontinuing an IV line.   When the radiographer must discontinue an IV line, the first step is handwashing. The following items are needed: a sterile adhesive bandage, scissors, and cotton balls or gauze sponges. The patient is then informed of what is to be done. Wearing gloves, the radiographer closes the drip control and gently removes the adhesive holding the catheter. (If it is necessary to cut the adhesive tape, take care not to cut the catheter because it may be doubled back under the tape.) This exposes the site where the catheter enters the vein. The catheter is removed in a long, smooth pull, and pressure is applied to the site with a cotton ball or sponge as soon as the needle is out. Pressure is maintained for a minute or until the bleeding stops. The site is then covered with a sterile adhesive bandage.

One reason for using a sterile cotton ball or sponge rather than an alcohol pledget is that the adhesive bandage is more likely to stick when dry pressure is used. Otherwise, one must wait until the alcohol has dried completely. After the patient is left in a safe, comfortable position, the equipment is disposed of in the proper container, gloves are removed, and the hands are washed again.

Precautions.   Most needles and syringes are provided in sterile wraps, used once, and then destroyed. One of the common on-the-job injuries in the past has been an accidental skin puncture by a contaminated needle. As discussed in Chapter 5, body substance precautions are essential for your safety as well as that of the patient. For this reason we strongly urge you to use caution.

1. Wear gloves when dealing with any object contaminated by blood or when inserting or removing an IV line.
2. Dispose of all syringes and needles directly into a puncture-proof container without recapping.
3. If absolutely necessary to recap a contaminated needle, place the cover on a firm surface and insert the needle using one hand only (Fig. 6-10), or use a needle cap holder.

Several additional points of critical importance must be remembered in all medication administration involving injections:

1. Always follow established rules of aseptic technique.
2. Read the label three times: before drawing up the medication, after drawing it up, and with the physician before administration.
3. Check patient identification before administration.
4. Monitor the patient carefully for side effects.

Monitoring IV fluids.   Patients who are receiving IV administration of fluids may come to the radiology department with a standard IV set or possibly a medication pump in place. Certain kidney diseases or cardiac problems may necessitate monitoring the patient's fluid intake very closely. For these patients, you must know how fast the IV set is supposed to run, not just how fast it was running when the patient entered the radiology department. Since these patients are almost always accompanied by their chart, look at the orders. If in doubt, call the floor nurse. Most patients easily tolerate 15 to 20 drops/minute from a standard IV set. At this rate the patient receives approximately 60 ml/hour. The drip rate is controlled by a clamp below the drip meter (Fig. 6-11),

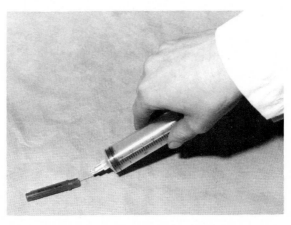

Fig. 6-10. Recap needles only when absolutely necessary; use one hand only.

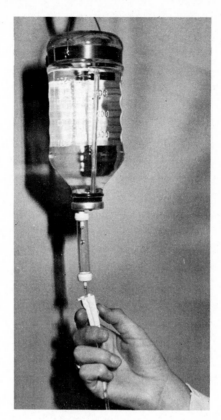

Fig. 6-11.   IV flow control. Practice improves precise regulation of drip rate.

which can be opened or closed to control the rate of flow. The radiographer should practice using this control in the laboratory before confronting it in the clinical area.

You may encounter an IV dripping slowly with a microdrip set (Fig. 6-12). The small size of the drops allows continuous flow at a reduced volume. This was once used extensively to keep an IV line open to administer medication. Although still used on occasion, especially for pediatric patients, intermittent injection ports have largely replaced "keep open" IV lines.

If an IV set runs too fast, a patient with chronic obstructive pulmonary disease or congestive heart failure may receive more fluid than can be readily assimilated, causing fluid to accumulate in the lungs (pulmonary edema). Since an IV set may also contain medication, the patient could suffer ill effects from too rapid administration. On the other hand, slow IV administration might cause inadequate medication dosage or prevent a contrast medium from being visualized effectively.

If you have changed the flow rate for any reason and are concerned about reregulating it correctly, be sure to call this to the attention of the nursing service when the patient is returned to their care.

In checking an IV set, you should remember several other precautions. Al-

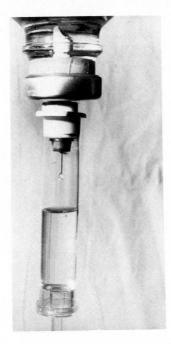

Fig. 6-12. Close-up view of microdrip chamber.

ways keep the IV solution 18 to 20 inches above the level of the vein. If the bottle is inadvertently placed lower than the vein, blood will flow back into the needle or tubing and may clot, causing the fluid to stop flowing. This frequently necessitates restarting the IV line at a new site. On the other hand, an IV solution that is too high may cause fluid to infiltrate into the surrounding tissues because of the increased hydrostatic pressure. Check the area around the injection site. If it is cool, swollen, and boggy, the IV solution may have infiltrated. In the case of infiltration, turn off the IV set and treat the area for extravasation as previously described.

Medication pumps (Fig. 6-13) are used for various reasons, including patient-controlled pain medication, parenteral nutrition, and continuous medication administration. If your clinical area deals frequently with patients on medication pumps, and especially if your work involves IV injections through lines governed by pumps, you must understand the operation of the specific pumps used in your facility. Medication pumps can be plugged into an electric outlet, but most pumps also have batteries that allow operation during transport. An alarm system is part of the pump and will emit a warning sound when the solution supply is low, when flow is interrupted, or when the battery power is weak. The ability to handle pumps competently are most easily acquired by hands-on practice under the direction of experienced personnel.

When a hanging supply of IV fluid is running low or when the pump alarm signals that an interruption in flow is imminent, one is strongly tempted to

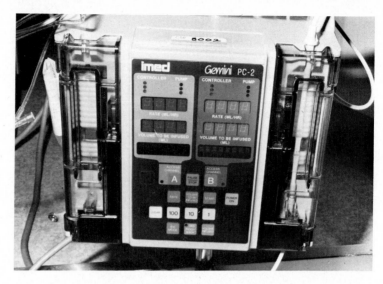

Fig. 6-13. IV pump governs infusions to regulate or permit self-administration of medication.

work rapidly, complete the procedure, and then return the patient promptly to the nursing service. All too often this results in a nonfunctioning or "blown" IV line. For some patients, starting a new IV line presents no particular problem. Unfortunately, patients who are hospitalized and receiving IV fluid or medication usually have the fewest suitable veins. This is particularly true of pediatric patients, whose tiny veins are both fragile and difficult to access. Patients receiving chemotherapy or parenteral nutrition are also likely to present difficulties when a new site is needed. You *can* avoid some of these problems by following these suggestions:

1. Call in advance and inform the medication nurse if the procedure will be lengthy.
2. Whenever possible, plug in the pump rather than relying on battery power.
3. Watch IV fluid levels and allow enough time for fluid replacement before the IV fluid is exhausted.
4. If an IV set does run out, or if the alarm sounds despite precautions, call the nursing service immediately rather than waiting until the patient is returned to the floor.

CHARTING MEDICATIONS

When a medication is given by a physician or by a radiographer under the physician's supervision, it is always recorded in the patient's chart. The notation is made in the appropriate section of the chart and includes the time of day, the name of the drug, the dosage, and the route of administration. A typical entry in the medication record might read: 10:50 AM, Benadryl, 50 mg, PO. Each entry must include the identification of the person who charted it. Initials alone are not considered to be adequate identification. If the medication record calls for initials, there is usually another place in the chart, often on the same page, where each set of initials is identified with the signer's full name. For legal purposes, the radiographer who charts medication must use the exact procedure established by the institution.

If an emergency prevents the charting of medications at the time they are given, the radiographer should make a written notation of the time, drug, and dosage so that accurate information will be available when the charting is completed. If this is not done, the pressure of the situation may lead to confusion of the facts, and the time, sequence, and dosage of several medications may be forgotten or charted incorrectly. Any medication prescribed or administered by a physician should be charted by the physician, or it should be countersigned by the physician if charted by the radiographer. The legal significance of complete accountability in such situations cannot be overemphasized.

The administration of contrast media is sometimes charted as a medication. More often, it is implied by the general charting of the examination and confirmed by a specific statement in the radiologist's report. If the latter method is employed, special notation may be required when there is a variation from the usual medium or dosage for a specific examination.

Although the physician may enter an account of the procedure and medication in the progress notes, the radiographer is responsible for checking that the drug, time, dose, and route of administration are clearly delineated for the nursing staff. In hospitals using problem-oriented medical recording (POMR), the radiographer may chart directly on progress notes; in other situations, it may be on the nurses' notes. Some hospitals have a medication administration sheet on which all medications must be charted. Charting routines vary. Familiarize yourself with the routine of your specific clinical area.

CONCLUSION

The radiographer is called on to play an important role in the administration of medications. Knowledge of common medications and their proper administration enables the radiographer to fulfill this role. Oral, topical, or parenteral medications may be administered in the radiology department, and each requires specialized knowledge and equipment. Intravenous access systems are used extensively in most hospitals and are the most frequent route of medication administration in imaging departments. The establishment of these systems, as well as their use and monitoring, requires that the radiographer have a high degree of knowledge, skill, and awareness.

The charting of medication and the monitoring of patients are significant aspects of medication administration and must not be overlooked. The radiographer must recognize the potential harm and legal complications that could result from medication administration errors and strive for error-free performance.

Study questions

1. Using the PDR, find two trade names for acetaminophen and the generic names for Valium and for Benadryl.
2. List two pairs of medication names that might be confused because they look or sound alike.
3. Under what circumstances might medication be given parenterally rather than orally?
4. Which route of medication administration has the highest potential for life-threatening side effects? Why?
5. Under what circumstances might a radiographer accept a verbal order from a physician? How should it be validated before the medication is administered?

Dealing with Acute Situations

Objectives

At the conclusion of this chapter, the student will be able to:

1. State the difference between syncope and vertigo.
2. Discuss seizure disorders, including safety precautions and observations to be recorded.
3. Demonstrate cardiopulmonary resuscitation, and state the code routine used by a specific clinical site.
4. Demonstrate the Heimlich maneuver.
5. List the four levels of consciousness.
6. Discuss the procedure for assisting a patient having an asthmatic attack, and state which medications are needed.
7. Describe the signs of physical and psychological shock.
8. List the precautions to be taken in handling fractures.
9. Contrast diabetic coma and insulin reaction or hypoglycemia.
10. Define *triage*.

Vocabulary list

1. cannula
2. cardiac arrest
3. comatose
4. concussion
5. COPD
6. crash cart
7. defibrillate
8. dehiscence
9. edema
10. epistaxis
11. evisceration
12. hemorrhage
13. ischemic
14. laceration
15. pleural effusion
16. pneumonia
17. tracheolaryngeal
18. tracheostomy
19. tremor
20. triage

An acute situation is any condition that causes a sudden deterioration in patient status. Whether such a situation leads to a more serious problem may depend on the radiographer's ability to respond quickly and appropriately. Seen from this perspective, *no patient problem is trivial*. You will encounter many acute situations and must be prepared to act in a way that will preserve life while minimizing the possibility of further injury or complication.

Although this chapter is basically organized to combine the discussion of acute situations with the correct methods for handling them, two procedures deserve special attention at the outset. Oxygen administration and the use of suction equipment are needed in a variety of acute situations.

OXYGEN ADMINISTRATION

You will often encounter patients who need supplemental oxygen. Oxygen may be prescribed to treat patients with traumatic respiratory problems or those with acute illnesses. It is always appropriate to provide oxygen to patients who experience anxiety accompanied by a rapid heart rate and shortness of breath.

Oxygen can be administered by mask, nasal cannula, or tent (Fig. 7-1). A nasal cannula is the simplest and most frequently used device. Always make certain that the oxygen is flowing through the cannula before placing it on the patient.

In most radiology departments, oxygen is available from a wall outlet, just as in most hospital acute care units. An oxygen flow gauge for a wall unit is shown in Fig. 7-2. The dial at the top is used to adjust the flow rate, which is indicated by the level of the ball shown near the bottom of the gauge.

During transport or in areas where oxygen is not otherwise available, portable oxygen units are used. The radiographer must be familiar with the operation of these units and with the procedure for checking to ensure that they will be available immediately when needed. The oxygen tank has an on-off valve that usually has a dial indicating how much gas remains (Fig. 7-3). The flow meter shows the rate at which oxygen is being delivered in units of liters per minute. Both valves must be turned on to provide oxygen to the patient.

The oxygen flow rate for many patients is 3 to 5 L/minute. Severely compromised patients, such as trauma victims in shock, may receive oxygen at a much higher rate. Patients with emphysema or chronic obstructive pulmonary disease (COPD) receive oxygen at a slower rate, less than 3 L/minute. These patients must not receive a higher rate of flow, since their rate of respiration is controlled by the level of carbon dioxide in the blood. If too much oxygen is administered, their respiratory rate may become too slow for adequate ventilation. If you are caring for a patient who is already receiving oxygen, note the rate of flow.

Remember that oxygen supports combustion, and care must be taken to prevent fire when oxygen is in use.

SUCTION

Mechanical suction is used to maintain the patient's airway by removing secretions, blood, or vomitus from the mouth and throat when the patient is unable

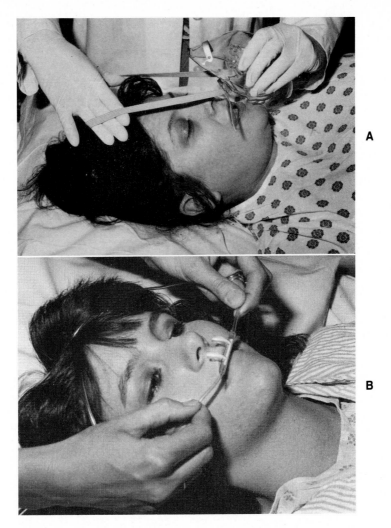

Fig. 7-1. Oxygen administration. **A,** Oxygen mask. **B,** Nasal cannula.

to do so. Many hospitals today have wall-mounted suction apparatus (Fig. 7-4), but some areas of the radiology department may still rely on movable machines. If suction procedures were not part of your orientation, you should assume responsibility for understanding and operating this equipment. Periodically check to ensure that the suction system is operational:

1. The pump is working.
2. The pump is properly connected to the receptacle.
3. An adequate length of plastic tubing leads from the receptacle.
4. A clean, disposable catheter is attached to the tubing and is covered to maintain cleanliness (sterility is not required).

Be alert to the need for suction whenever a patient becomes nauseated, is bleeding from the mouth or nose, or is unable to swallow and cope with secre-

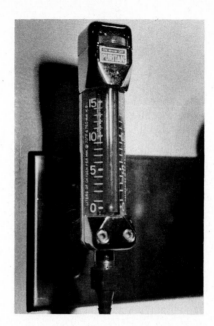

Fig. 7-2. Oxygen gauge on wall outlet system.

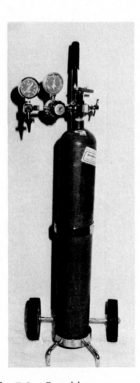

Fig. 7-3. Portable oxygen unit.

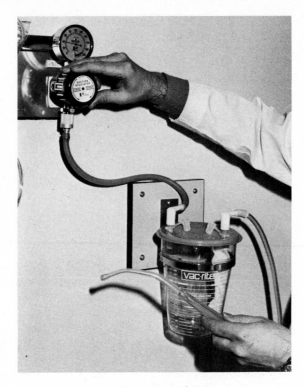

Fig. 7-4. Wall-mounted suction apparatus.

tions because of a low level of consciousness. If a patient does aspirate mucus or vomitus, turn the patient immediately to the lateral recumbent position, don a glove, and attempt to clear the airway manually. Remember to stand aside when clearing an airway, since the sudden violent expulsion of the obstructing material may spray into your face. If a reflex cough does not occur at this point, suction may be needed.

It would be unusual for a radiographer to work alone with an unconscious patient who is likely to aspirate. Such patients are usually accompanied by a nurse or physician, and your role is to assist in the procedure. Unwrap the suction tip attached to the suction apparatus, and turn on the suction. At this point the nurse proceeds with suctioning while you assist by holding the patient in position. When the emergency is over, check to be sure that you have cleaned or replaced the receptacle and replaced the disposable tip and tubing so that the suction unit will be ready for use when needed.

In the event that you must suction the patient yourself, use your emergency call button or call for help while you unwrap the catheter and turn on the suction. After you have cleared the mouth, pull the chin down and forward while inserting the suction catheter tip over the tongue in the midline. Do not insert the catheter forcibly, since you may injure the larynx. Any suctioning beyond the nasopharynx should be done by a physician or someone trained in this procedure.

LIFE-THREATENING EMERGENCIES

An emergency is a condition or sudden change in a patient's status that requires immediate attention. Since radiographic studies are often necessary for the evaluation of emergencies, the radiographer may expect to encounter these situations. When care is given in the radiology department, the patient's condition is usually stable enough to permit transportation without undue risk. Occasionally, however, a life-threatening situation may develop. In this event the three objectives of the radiographer are to preserve life, prevent further problems, and obtain medical help as quickly as possible. The process of obtaining help will vary depending on your situation. When other team members are nearby, use a loud, firm voice to call for a specific person by name, for example, "Dr. Logan, please come to Room 3 immediately." Your control over the situation is reassuring to the patient and will be likely to result in a more positive form of assistance than a bleat of "Help!"

Emergency call systems

When working alone or when qualified assistance is not immediately available, use the emergency call system. Each hospital has a procedure to call for emergency help, and usually several specific codes are available depending on the situation. The fire code mentioned in Chapter 3 is one example. Other codes may be used to summon help for the patient undergoing cardiopulmonary arrest, to announce the arrival of trauma patients in the emergency department, or to cope with a situation that demands security personnel. Whatever system is used, be completely familiar with it. Practice going through a code until you feel comfortable with the entire procedure.

Emergency carts

Emergency carts, or "crash carts," are rolling, multidrawered cabinets that are kept in strategic locations throughout the hospital (Fig. 7-5). The code team usually brings the cart from the location nearest the patient. These carts vary somewhat, but each has certain essential items, such as airways, artificial ventilation equipment, emergency medications and the equipment for administering them, a board to slip under the patient when giving external cardiac massage, a blood pressure cuff, a stethoscope, and a defibrillator, which can serve as a cardiac monitor. The cart should have a list of contents and be inspected daily to ensure that all emergency supplies are available for instant use. Some hospitals seal the cart after supplies are replenished. Never borrow equipment or supplies from the emergency set for routine use. This practice results in the absence of lifesaving items when they are most needed.

Table 7-1 lists typical medications found on an emergency cart and can help you become familiar with common emergency drugs and their actions. Learn both the proprietary (trade) and generic names. If a drug should be called for by trade name and the emergency stock is the generic equivalent by a different manufacturer, you must be able to identify the correct medication by the generic name. This table is not meant to be a substitute for thorough knowledge of the contents of the emergency cart in your clinical setting.

Some emergency carts contain bags of intravenous (IV) solutions to which

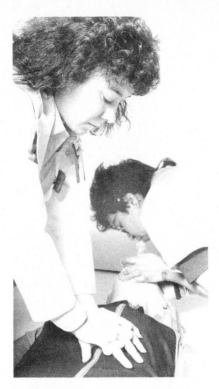

Fig. 7-6. Students practice CPR on resuscitation dummy. Person doing external cardiac massage needs to keep her fingers up.

mally. They may have learned esophageal speech (the ability to swallow air and form words while belching it back), or they may use an artificial external larynx. Care must be taken not to obstruct the airway. If the patient with a tracheostomy undergoes cardiopulmonary arrest, you must ventilate through the tracheostomy when doing CPR. Place your mouth tightly over the opening and blow, using the same timing as in regular CPR.

Once the code team has arrived, you may no longer feel needed, but a radiographer can perform several important tasks. Record keeping is essential. Write down the time the attack started and when the code team responded. You may be asked to record times and amounts of medications or when defibrillation was administered. It may be necessary to obtain equipment, call for other personnel, or monitor a telephone.

When a code is initiated, your help may be needed to connect the patient to the cardiac monitor (Fig. 7-7). The monitor is connected by means of electrical leads that snap onto adhesive disks attached to the patient's upper torso. The wire leads and adhesive pads are stored with the monitor. Know how to check the monitor and the related supplies in your area. You may need to know how to connect a patient to the monitor, print a tape of the monitor reading, and change the tape when necessary. Since cardiac monitors vary, use of this equipment should be part of your in-service instruction.

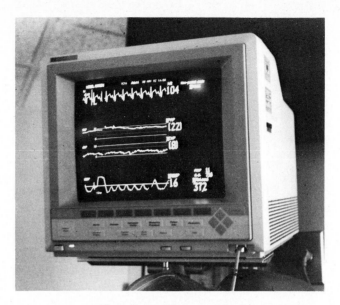

Fig. 7-7. Cardiac monitor.

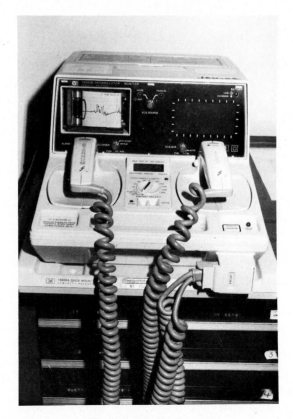

Fig. 7-8. Defibrillator.

With the help of the cardiac monitor, the code team may determine that the *defibrillator* (Fig. 7-8) is needed. This machine administers an electric shock to correct an ineffectual cardiac rhythm. The defibrillator does not need to be plugged in, since it has an auxiliary battery system for use beyond the reach of electrical outlets. It must be turned on and set at the proper voltage. Two paddles attached to the machine make contact with the patient's chest. The paddle surfaces must be covered with disposable pads to protect the skin and facilitate the electrical contact. When the equipment and the team are ready, CPR is interrupted, and the word "Clear" is used to signal caution before the shock. This is a warning to stand clear of the patient, the bed, or anything connected to the patient. A 2-foot distance is adequate. If the first shock is not successful, defibrillation may be repeated.

Respiratory arrest

Respiratory arrest may occur in the absence of cardiac arrest or any cardiac problem. It can be caused by localized swelling in the upper respiratory tract, failure of the central nervous system (CNS), or choking on a foreign object. Tracheolaryngeal edema can be severe enough to cause respiratory arrest. The swelling may be very rapid, as in an allergic response to the injection of iodinated contrast media, or more gradual, as in an infectious process. If the edema is sufficient to prevent respiration, it may be necessary to perform an emergency tracheotomy. In this procedure, an artificial opening is made into the trachea to allow ventilation. Because the potential for allergic reaction exists with IV contrast studies, a tracheotomy tray is frequently kept in the radiology department. If not, one should be found on the emergency cart. Since this tray is used so seldom, be sure to check the sterilization date regularly.

Respiratory arrest caused by CNS failure is usually associated with an overdose of medication, misuse of a controlled substance, or a severe head injury. These patients usually require intubation and artificial ventilation and are seen most often in the intensive care unit (ICU).

Respiratory arrest may also result from a blocked airway caused by aspiration of foreign material (choking). In this event, don a glove and clear the airway manually. If this is unsuccessful, proceed with suction, as described previously, while calling for assistance. If respiration has not resumed and you are trained in CPR, the next step is to administer an abdominal thrust in an attempt to dislodge the foreign material.

Sudden respiratory arrest from any cause is a life-threatening problem. An emergency code should be called.

A common example of respiratory arrest caused by choking occurs when an older person enjoying a festive meal has difficulty chewing the meat. To avoid embarrassment, the meat may be swallowed whole and lodge at the larynx. The combination of alcohol, talking while eating, and poorly fitting dentures predisposes to such a "café coronary," which is not a "heart attack" at all.

When a foreign body lodges in the opening of the trachea, people frequently become quite agitated, their faces become congested, and they may tear at their collars or throats. Since the lungs hold more air than is normally used during respiration, the reserve supply can be used to help dislodge a foreign body, us-

Fig. 7-9.

Heimlich maneuver for choking persons.

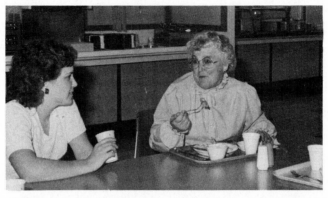

Choking is most common among older persons enjoying a meal.

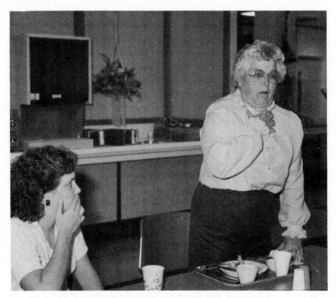

Choking person becomes agitated, cannot speak,
and tears at throat; face is congested.

Fig. 7-9.   **Heimlich maneuver for choking persons—cont'd.**

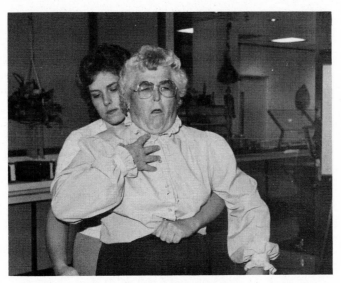

Stand behind victim. Place fist in middle of abdomen
with thumb just below ribs.

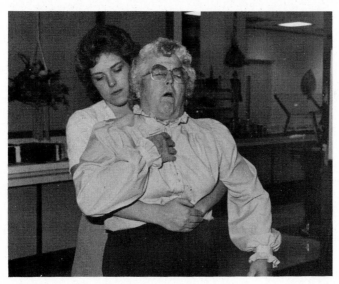

Grasp wrist with other hand. Apply quick, forceful pressure
upward against diaphragm to compress lungs and expel aspirated object.

ing a technique called the *Heimlich maneuver*. Ask, "Can you speak?" If the person does not answer, stand behind him or her and place both arms around the waist, with one hand grasping the opposite wrist. Quickly and *forcefully* apply pressure upward against the diaphragm just below the ribs. This will compress the lungs and expel the aspirated object (Fig. 7-9).

Shock

Shock is a general term used to describe a failure of circulation in which blood pressure is inadequate to support oxygen perfusion of vital tissues and is unable to remove the by-products of metabolism. Shock is a dangerous, potentially fatal condition. There are five main types of shock:

1. *Hypovolemic shock* occurs when such a large amount of blood or plasma has been lost that an insufficient amount of fluid is available to fill the circulatory system. This may result from external hemorrhage, lacerations, or plasma loss from burns. Internal bleeding, such as that into the peritoneum from a perforated gastric ulcer, can also cause shock. Low-volume shock is treated by fluid replacement.

2. *Septic shock* occurs when a massive infection, such as one caused by gram-negative bacteria, produces toxins, causing the blood pressure to drop sharply. In addition to antibiotic therapy, emergency treatment for the shock itself must be initiated immediately (see following information).

3. *Neurogenic shock,* the failure of arterial resistance, causes a pooling of blood in peripheral vessels. It occurs in reaction to an injury to the nervous system and is an acute situation that demands immediate, drastic intervention. Patients with head or spinal trauma must be monitored closely for a decrease in blood pressure.

4. *Cardiogenic shock* results from cardiac failure or interference with heart function. A pulmonary embolus or a reaction to anesthesia may initiate such an event. In trauma patients, cardiac tamponade may be the precipitating factor. This occurs when a blow to the chest results in the pericardium (sac around heart) being filled with blood. The resulting pressure interferes with the heart's pumping ability.

5. *Allergic shock,* or *anaphylaxis,* occurs when individuals receive injections of foreign protein to which they are sensitized. An allergic reaction develops, which affects blood vessels and other tissues directly. Blood pressure falls rapidly, severe dyspnea caused by respiratory obstruction from edema may develop, and death can result if this is not recognized and treated rapidly. Bee stings and injections of certain medications, including iodinated contrast media, are the most common causes of anaphylactic reaction. In the radiology department, this will most likely occur during or immediately after the injection of contrast media.

The following symptoms indicate some degree of shock in any or all combinations:

1. Restlessness and a sense of apprehension
2. Increased pulse rate
3. Pallor accompanied by weakness or a change in thinking ability
4. Cool, clammy skin (except in patients with septic or neurogenic shock)

  5. A fall in blood pressure of 30 mm below the baseline systolic pressure

Your responsibility to patients with any type of shock is to recognize symptoms of impending shock, to know the location of emergency medical supplies, and to be thoroughly familiar with the code routine of your institution. The physician may call on your knowledge of medications and your medication administration skills during treatment. The radiographer's role in suspected shock is as follows:

  1. Stop the procedure.
  2. Protect the patient from falling by assisting him or her to lie in a dorsal recumbent position with the feet elevated.
  3. Obtain help. If in doubt, call a code. It is much better to be mistaken than to have a patient die because of inadequate treatment.
  4. Check blood pressure.
  5. Assist the dyspneic patient with oxygen.
  6. Be ready to perform CPR.
  7. Assist the code team or physician as necessary.
  8. Chart the occurrence, the treatment administered, and the patient's response on an incident report form or in the chart.

Trauma

Many hospitals have specialized facilities designated as *trauma units,* which may be part of the emergency department. These are designed to cope with massive, life-threatening injuries. Many units have the resources to accept patients who have been airlifted directly to the unit from a considerable distance. Trauma physicians receive highly specialized training in the diagnosis and treatment of traumatic injury. Although the composition may vary slightly, the staff usually consists of one or more physicians, trauma nurses, anesthetist or respiratory therapist, radiographer(s), phlebotomist, and one individual (who may also be a nurse) to act as record keeper. Research has proved that patients with massive trauma who survive the initial injury have a greater chance of recovery if their condition can be stabilized within the first "golden" hour after the accident. For this reason, every minute is precious, and trauma teams work under great pressure.

The transport team, usually paramedics, delivers the patient as soon as they have established an airway, controlled bleeding, and immobilized the patient. One of the first assessments made by the physician at the trauma unit is the possibility of vertebral fracture. Trauma patients are transported on a rigid backboard and are not removed from it until spinal fracture has been ruled out. The danger of paralysis is so great that this ranks directly after respiratory and cardiac arrest in terms of priority.

The radiographic protocols usually state that lateral cervical spine and chest films should be taken on all trauma patients. The cassettes for radiographs of the cervical spine, chest, and pelvis should be present in each mobile unit to avoid delays. In addition to mobile x-ray and possibly C-arm fluoroscopic units, many trauma areas also have a computed tomography (CT) scanner and small surgical suite immediately adjacent. The highly trained personnel and the immediate availability of equipment for diagnosis and treatment have greatly improved the potential for saving the lives of patients with massive trauma.

By the time most victims of accidents arrive in the radiology department, their conditions have usually been stabilized. They have been thoroughly examined by a physician, blood loss has been controlled, an airway has been established, IV fluids have been started, if necessary, and medication for pain or blood pressure control has been given. When radiographs are taken en route to the operating room, cast room, or intensive care unit, the patient is frequently accompanied by a nurse.

Emergency patients are subject to sudden changes in condition and may go into physical or psychological shock. Once the acute phase of an accident is over, many patients who were full of fortitude experience a delayed emotional reaction. This may take the form of uncontrollable crying or a compulsive urge to tell everyone about the accident. They may even have a physical reaction, such as fainting, trembling, or violent nausea. Your most positive action is to be available, offer nonverbal support, and watch carefully for any signs of deteriorating physical condition. Your ability to speak calmly and work competently under pressure is reassuring.

When trauma patients are still dressed in street clothes, it is sometimes necessary to remove garments before the radiographic examination. Avoid cutting or tearing clothing whenever possible. Keep all the patient's personal possessions together in one place. One easy system is to place everything in a plastic bag clearly identified with the patient's name. The bag is then placed on the stretcher or wheelchair with the patient. Check the procedure in your clinical area and be consistent in using it.

Head injuries

Patients who have received a blow to the head may have sustained serious injury, even when no external signs of trauma are present. Damage may occur with or without a skull fracture. The brain is soft, has a rich blood supply, and is suspended in cerebrospinal fluid within the skull. A severe blow to the head causes the brain to bounce from side to side, resulting in injury on the side opposite the blow. This is usually called *contrecoup* damage. A minimal amount of damage, characterized by "seeing stars" or very brief loss of consciousness, is called a *concussion*. If bleeding or swelling occurs inside the skull, a rise in intracranial pressure (ICP) may cause seizures, respiratory arrest, or loss of consciousness. Brain tumors may also result in increased ICP, causing patients to exhibit similar symptoms.

Four levels of consciousness are generally recognized and may be described as (1) alert and conscious; (2) drowsy, but responsive; (3) unconscious, but reactive to painful stimuli; and (4) comatose. The patient who is alert and oriented when admitted, then becomes increasingly incoherent, drowsy, and stuporous, may be showing signs of increased ICP. The earliest signs of increasing pressure may be irritability and lethargy, frequently associated with a slowing pulse and slow respirations. Notify the attending physician immediately if you suspect a change in level of consciousness. Remember that the unconscious patient must have side rails in place, should not be left alone, and must be constantly monitored to maintain an airway.

Fig. 7-10.   **"Logrolling" procedure for patient with spinal injury.**

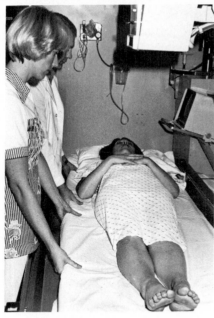

By pulling table pad toward you as you roll patient in one plane, patient remains centered to table.

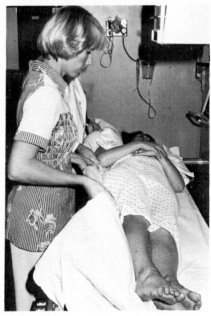

Take care that spine does not bend or twist. Note position of patient's hands.

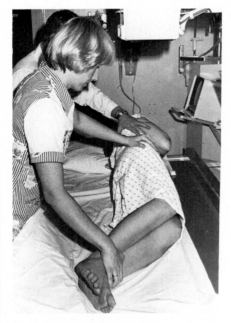

As you near lateral position, place hand on patient for safety. Flexing knees helps to maintain this position.

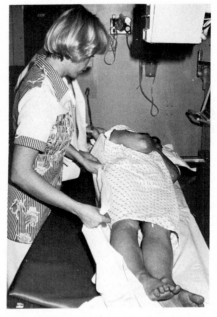

The sheet alone may serve as support for returning patient to supine position.

Some trauma patients are under the influence of alcohol. Their condition may vary from inappropriate jocularity to an alcoholic stupor, or they may be argumentative or verbally abusive. It is easy to assume that the unconscious intoxicated patient has "passed out" because of a high level of blood alcohol, but these patients are as subject to sudden changes in condition as nonintoxicated persons. It is just as important to be alert to levels of consciousness in these patients as in others with head injuries. Patients taking pain medications or diabetic patients who are insulin dependent and have gone too long without insulin may show similar signs and symptoms.

Spinal injuries

Every trauma patient should be considered to have a potential spinal injury and should be evaluated by a physician before being moved. Even slight movement of a spinal fracture may cause pressure on the spinal cord, resulting in paralysis or death. For this reason, exposures should be made without moving the patient whenever possible. When a change of position is required, as for a lateral lumbar radiograph, use a "logrolling" approach, which keeps the body in one plane and avoids twisting or bending the spine (Fig. 7-10).

Patients with possible cervical spine fractures are immobilized with cervical collars and other radiolucent devices. These must remain in place during initial radiographic examinations and until a physician has determined that it is safe for them to be removed. A cross-table lateral radiograph of the cervical-spine is taken with the mobile unit and evaluated before moving the patient from the backboard or ambulance stretcher.

Extremity fractures

Trauma involving the long bones of the body may be classified in two categories: (1) compound fractures, in which the splintered ends of bone are forced through the skin, and (2) closed fractures. Compound fractures are usually partially reduced, with a dressing applied before radiographic examination. Fractures may also be classified according to the nature of the injury. Some common fracture types are illustrated in Fig. 7-11.

There are many ways of temporarily immobilizing fractures. The two legs may be fastened together for stability during transportation (self-splinting), or a stiff object, such as a board or rolled-up magazine, may serve as a splint. Ambulances often carry pneumatic splints, which are essentially air-filled sleeves that protect and immobilize the extremity (Fig. 7-12). Splinting devices should not be removed except under the physician's direct supervision.

When you must position a fractured extremity that is not supported by a splint, maintain gentle traction while supporting and moving the arm or leg. Two people may be required to support and position patients with a potential long bone fracture, since the extremity must be supported at sites both proximal and distal to the injury. It is important to minimize motion of the fracture fragments. This helps avoid unnecessary pain and, more importantly, the initiation of a muscle spasm, which could interfere with the physician's attempt to reduce and immobilize the fracture more permanently. Movement of fracture fragments may also tear surrounding soft tissues, nerves, and blood vessels.

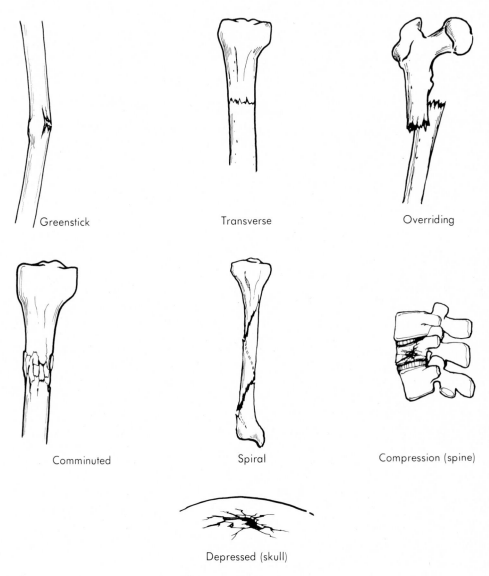

Greenstick   Transverse   Overriding

Comminuted   Spiral   Compression (spine)

Depressed (skull)

Fig. 7-11. Fracture types.

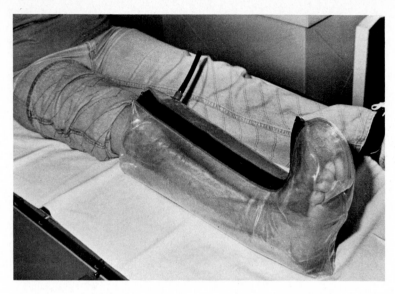

Fig. 7-12. Pneumatic splint for lower leg.

Special care is required when positioning extremities following application of a plaster cast. Undue pressure against a fresh (wet) cast may cause it to change shape. Lift the casted extremity by placing your open hands underneath it; never grasp it from above. Observe the fingers or toes for evidence of impaired circulation. They should be warm, pink, and sensitive to touch and pressure. Coldness, numbness, or lack of normal coloration should be reported to the physician at once.

Wounds

Patients with open wounds usually have been treated before you see them in the radiology suite. Bleeding has been controlled and a dressing applied. The radiographer's primary responsibility regarding open wounds is to maintain the dressings and to report promptly any significant amount of fresh bleeding, that is, an amount of bright-red blood sufficient to soak through a fresh dressing. If a laceration or incision opens, causing severe hemorrhaging, apply direct pressure to the site of bleeding while summoning immediate assistance.

Burns

Burns do not usually require radiographic evaluation but are frequently associated with respiratory complications as well as other traumatic injuries, such as fractures. Inhalation of hot gases may result in pleural effusion or the development of pneumonia, which must be monitored radiographically. If a burn patient needs to be moved, coordinate your examination with the nursing staff to ensure that the patient has had pain medication about 30 minutes before the procedure. If the patient is under protective precautions, you may wish to review this technique (see Chapter 5).

Burn patients may have grafts or healing skin that is extremely tender. Such tissue is easily damaged during transfers or positioning; therefore you should allow patients to move themselves as much as possible. If necessary, ask for help and use a sheet to avoid abrasion.

MEDICAL EMERGENCIES

Nausea

Nausea and vomiting are frequently encountered, and a well-prepared radiographer learns to cope easily with this situation. Occasionally, patients may feel nauseated for a specific reason, such as after swallowing a barium preparation. Vomiting can often be prevented by the radiographer's reassuring touch and presence and by the instruction to "Breathe through your mouth, taking short, rapid, panting breaths." On the other hand, if a patient expresses a need for an emesis basin, offer it immediately. Provide tissues and water to rinse the mouth. It is especially important to support the patient in a sitting or lateral recumbent position to avoid aspiration of vomitus. If the patient loses consciousness, be sure to turn the head to the side and clear the airway. Bring the patient a clean emesis basin before removing the soiled one.

Reactions to contrast media

Intravascular agents require special precautions because adverse reactions may occur. Radiographers must be alert to observe the onset of these reactions and be prepared to deal with them when they occur. Possible adverse effects include mild to severe nausea, urticaria or "hives" (blotchy reddening of the skin with itching), asthmatic attack, laryngeal edema, anaphylactic shock, and cardiac arrest. About 5% of patients have some adverse reaction, and about 5% of those who react demonstrate a severe or life-threatening response. The causes of these reactions have been studied at length but are still unknown. However, the reactions have been shown *not* to result from antibody formation, which is the usual cause of allergic response.

If reaction symptoms are minor, such as nausea, vomiting, flushing, or coughing, little treatment is needed. Provide an emesis basin, alert the radiologist, and continue to observe the patient carefully. An intermediate reaction is characterized by erythema (reddening of the skin), urticaria (hives), or asthma. The treatment for these patients is administration of an antihistamine medication, such as diphenhydramine (Benadryl), either intravenously or intramuscularly, depending on the reaction's severity. Some physicians prefer to give epinephrine at this point.

A severe reaction is called *anaphylactic shock.* It is a life-threatening condition that may result in respiratory or cardiac arrest. The early symptoms of anaphylaxis include a sense of warmth, tingling, itching of palms and soles, dysphagia (difficulty swallowing), constriction in the throat, a feeling of doom, an expiratory wheeze, and then progression into laryngeal and bronchial edema. The treatments for shock, respiratory arrest, and cardiac arrest are outlined elsewhere in this chapter. At the onset of anaphylaxis the radiographer should maintain the patient's airway, alert the radiologist, and call a code.

Although most reactions occur almost immediately, delayed responses may be seen and should be anticipated for at least 30 minutes after the injection. In rare instances, reactions have occurred as long as several hours after the injection. Interestingly, patients do not experience allergic reactions when under general anesthesia. One investigator, Dr. A.F. Lalli, has demonstrated a connection between anxiety and adverse reactions. He speculated that the deterrent effect of antihistamine drugs may be caused as much by the soporific (causing sleep) effect of the antihistamine as by its specific action. To alleviate anxiety as a factor in potential adverse reactions, one must provide the patient with a reasonable explanation of what to expect without causing alarm. Most patients experience a feeling of warmth during injection and may feel flushed for 1 to 3 minutes afterward. An unusual "metallic" taste is often reported, and a brief period of nausea also frequently occurs. This passes quickly and does not usually produce vomiting if the patient is relaxed.

Asthma

Asthma is difficulty in breathing caused by bronchospasm. Asthmatic attacks are frequently precipitated by stress, and if the radiologic procedure is new or frightening, dyspnea may result. The usual response to respiratory distress is to administer oxygen, but this is *not* the treatment of choice for patients with asthma. The objective is to relieve the bronchospasm. Most chronic asthmatic persons carry a nebulizer with a bronchodilating medication. Patients with asthma should take their medication into the examining room. For an acute episode, the treatment is an injection of epinephrine, which is ordered by the physician. Although anxiety producing to both patient and radiographer, a single asthmatic attack is seldom fatal.

Heart attack

If a patient complains of sudden, intense chest pain, often described as a crushing pain, you should assume that the patient may be having a heart attack until proved otherwise. Since the pain is caused when a portion of the heart wall becomes ischemic, you must prevent further damage by minimizing patient exertion. Patients may underestimate the importance of this type of pain and assume instead that the sudden onset is "terrible heartburn" or "indigestion from that peanut butter sandwich." These patients often become diaphoretic and pale and may feel nauseated. Stay with the patient, *obtain help,* and assist the patient to a comfortable position. If the patient has shortness of breath, raise the head and administer oxygen.

Syncope

Syncope, or fainting, is a very mild form of neurogenic shock that sometimes occurs with fright, pain, or unpleasant events that are beyond the coping ability of the patient's nervous system. Blood pressure falls as the diameter of the blood vessels increases and the heart rate slows. When the blood pressure is too low to supply the brain with oxygen, the patient faints. Placing the patient in a dorsal recumbent position with the feet elevated usually relieves this type of shock. Patients who have been NPO for 12 hours and are feeling anxious and stressed may undergo syncope. Patients who feel faint should be assisted into a sitting or recumbent position. If a chair is not within reach, ease the patient to the floor. If the patient does not rouse immediately, spirits of ammonia held under the nose usually cause a rapid return to consciousness. Small, crushable vials of ammonia are usually kept in the radiology department for this purpose. Anyone who has more than a momentary loss of consciousness should be evaluated by a physician before the examination is resumed.

Postural hypotension and vertigo

A lightheaded or dizzy sensation is not unusual after prolonged bed rest; postural hypotension is the usual cause. This results from the same basic mechanism as that causing syncope. Blood pools in the extremities when the torso is elevated and causes a transient cerebral anoxia. This condition can usually be avoided by having the patient sit up gradually. This sensation frequently affects elderly patients, so remain close to them and provide support when a sudden change in position is necessary.

Vertigo has a different cause. The patient does not feel "lightheaded" but describes the *room* as moving or whirling. These patients frequently cling to the table and will fall if not assisted to lie down. They may experience violent nausea. This sensation is usually attributed to either a middle ear disturbance or a lesion in the brain or spinal cord. Alcohol or drugs may affect certain individuals in a similar manner. If the onset is sudden and the patient does not have a previous history of vertigo, you may need to consult the physician before proceeding.

Wound dehiscence

Patients who have extensive abdominal surgery may require radiographic examination. If they are ambulatory or assist themselves onto the table, stand by to steady them and ensure against a fall. Wound dehiscence and possible evisceration result when sutures spread apart or split. This may occur when infection has weakened the tissues or when an obese patient experiences a sudden strain, such as a fall; a severe attack of coughing; or vomiting. The patient may tell you that something has given way and may complain of pain, or a rush of liquid may saturate the dressings. If this should occur, ease the patient to a sitting position and summon a physician immediately.

Unless specific orders exist to the contrary, leave abdominal binders in place during the examination, since these supports help prevent such an occurrence. If you must remove the binder, wait until the patient is comfortably situated on the radiographic table. Replace the binder before the patient is transferred back to the stretcher or wheelchair.

Seizures

Patients with seizure disorders are often seen in the radiology department for examinations such as a skull series, a cerebral arteriogram, or a CT scan. In the event of a seizure, your first duty is to keep the patient as safe as possible. A major motor (or grand mal) seizure may be preceded by an aura or premonitory sign. The patient may say, "I'm going to have a spell." Frequently the seizure is signaled by a hoarse cry when air is forced past the vocal cords by a sudden contraction of all the abdominal and chest muscles. Assist the patient to lie down. Remove any objects that might be hazardous, and place padding under the patient's head. Do not attempt to restrain the patient. Loss of consciousness and a rigid arching of the back are followed by alternate relaxation and rigidity of the muscles until the seizure passes and the patient slowly regains consciousness. While unconscious, involuntary voiding may occur. In the immediate (postictal) period following the seizure, the patient may be somewhat irritable or confused and wish only to sleep.

Less intense motor seizures may cause severe, uncontrollable tremors. This condition often causes extreme anxiety and hyperventilation in a conscious patient. These seizures are exhausting to the patient and may persist for over an hour without treatment. Notify a physician immediately. Stand by to reassure the patient and have Valium ready for administration. Instruct the patient to breathe slowly, and place a paper bag over nose and mouth if hyperventilation is otherwise uncontrollable.

Another type of seizure is characterized by a brief loss of consciousness (absence) during which the patient stares or may lose balance and fall. Many patients are not aware that they undergo this loss of consciousness.

Patients taking anticonvulsant medication may not have seizures for long periods. Most of these medications have a relatively slow excretion rate, which allows the patient to miss a dose or two without precipitating an attack. On the other hand, fatigue, apprehension, and the demands of a rigorous preparation for examination may initiate a seizure in a previously stable patient.

Realize that the seizure will run its course. The most important actions you can take are protect the patient from harm and be an accurate observer. Note when the seizure began and how long it lasted. Did it involve both sides of the body equally, and did the contractions start in one area and progress from one extremity to another? These observations can be helpful to the physician in reaching an accurate diagnosis.

Remember that not all seizure-prone individuals have the same diagnosis. Seizures may be a response to drug sensitivity, infection, epilepsy, tumor, or fever. Only recently have the old superstitions and myths about seizure disorders begun to be dispelled. No direct, consistent correlation exists between seizures and mental acuity, emotional instability, or heredity.

Alcoholics who are hospitalized for medical treatment do not always reveal the extent of their addiction to their physicians. After 48 hours, they may have withdrawal symptoms, including visual and auditory hallucinations and tremors. Some also experience major motor seizures.

Epistaxis

A nosebleed, or epistaxis, is rather frightening to the patient but is usually not serious. Remove eyeglasses, when necessary, and provide an ample supply of tissues. Instruct the patient to breathe through the mouth and to squeeze firmly against the nasal septum for 10 minutes. The patient should *not* lie down, blow the nose, or talk. Provide an emesis basin, instructing the patient to spit out blood that runs down the nasopharynx rather than swallow it. If bleeding lasts more than a few minutes, inform the physician, who may want to apply more direct treatment.

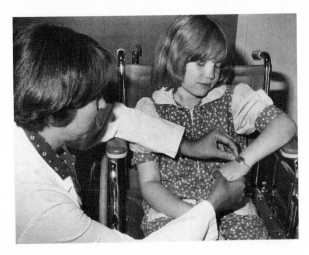

Fig. 7-13. Medic-Alert bracelet identifies diabetic patient.

Diabetic coma and insulin reactions

Patients who have diabetes are seen for the same problems that bring other patients to the radiology department. Since diabetes is sometimes associated with circulatory problems, these patients may be candidates for arteriograms as well as for more routine procedures. The diabetic patient can often be identified by means of the Medic-Alert bracelet (Fig. 7-13). (These bracelets are also worn by persons with other medical conditions that may require emergency treatment. The nature of the problem is stated on the bracelet and can be of great help in providing an appropriate emergency response.)

Diabetes is a disease characterized by an inability to metabolize blood glucose. Insulin is an enzyme normally produced in the pancreas in response to food intake. Insufficient insulin prevents the use of glucose by the muscles. When the muscles cannot use glucose, the liver forms ketone bodies to supply energy to the muscles. When excess ketone bodies appear in the blood, ketoacidosis develops. The body attempts to compensate for the acidosis by hyperventilation (air hunger) and the loss of minerals and water in the urine. When the blood glucose level is very high, sugar also spills over into the urine. The individual who is terribly thirsty, urinates copious amounts frequently, and has fruity smelling breath may be approaching diabetic coma. This condition is characterized by a relatively *slow onset.* The patient is diagnosed through blood and urine tests and treated with diet, exercise, and medication, such as insulin or hypoglycemic agents.

The diabetic patient who has taken insulin but no food may develop *hypoglycemia,* or *low blood sugar.* This is characterized by the *sudden onset* of weakness, sweating, tremors, hunger, and finally, loss of consciousness. While the patient is still alert and cooperative, hypoglycemia can be quickly remedied by administration of a small amount of candy or sweet fruit juice. Many departments have squeeze tubes containing a measured amount of glucose with the emer-

---

Characteristics of impending diabetic crisis

Hyperglycemia	Hypoglycemia
High blood sugar	Low blood sugar
Flushed, dry skin and mucous membranes	Sweating, clammy, cold skin
Air hunger with fruity smelling breath	Nervousness and irritability
Excessive thirst and urination	Blurred vision
Slow onset	Rapid onset

---

gency medications. These prepackaged tubes are useful in that the gel-like material can be placed inside the patient's cheek, which decreases the chance that a semiconscious or confused patient will aspirate candy or juice.

Report the occurrence of such symptoms to the physician. You must help these patients to sit or lie down until the sugar takes effect. Occasionally, individuals with the same symptoms may be adamant that they do not have diabetes. They may have hypoglycemia without diabetes; the treatment is the same. The box above summarizes the physical findings associated with both high blood sugar, indicative of approaching diabetic coma, and low blood sugar, which may signify an impending insulin reaction.

MULTIPLE EMERGENCIES

Up to this point, it has been assumed that the radiographer will encounter only one emergency at a time. Often, however, a single accident will have multiple victims or two or more acute situations will develop simultaneously. In these cases, you must assess priorities. If you see that it may be difficult for you to cope alone, do not hesitate to call for assistance *before* the situation becomes life-threatening.

Although patients are usually admitted to the radiology department on a scheduled or first come/first served basis, exceptions must obviously be made for emergencies. An order designated "stat" is to be done *at once* and indicates that the patient's well-being may be seriously jeopardized by any delay. When more than one patient from the emergency department requires examination at the same time, the radiographer may need to determine which patient's status is the most urgent. Generally, the highest priority is assigned to patients whose vital signs are unstable and whose immediate care depends on the results of the examination, such as those in severe respiratory distress. With two cases of apparently equal urgency, start with the patient who can be examined in the shortest time, since this decision will result in the shortest total waiting period.

On rare occasions, a major accident such as a plane crash or train wreck will result in many victims to be cared for at the same time. These events are properly termed "disasters." All general hospitals are required to have a carefully designed and written "disaster plan," and each member of the health care team must be familiar with the plan and his or her role in it. Disaster drills are regularly scheduled exercises that prepare the hospital staff to function effectively in the event that the disaster plan must be implemented. The radiographer must be familiar with the plan for the institution and participate attentively in the practice drills.

Although disaster plans differ somewhat, depending on the hospital, certain elements are usually similar. A single person is designated to be responsible for the overall implementation of the plan. This person is notified immediately of the nature and scope of the disaster and evaluates the need for additional personnel, coordinating activities with other institutions and governmental agencies as needed. A special communications network, established in advance, is used to notify all needed personnel who are not on duty. This system usually consists of a series of telephone calls, with each person called contacting three or four others before leaving home for the hospital. This method provides rapid notification to many people without jamming the hospital telephone lines.

The process of identifying the victims, performing initial examinations, and assigning priorities for further care is called *triage*. A triage station is set up in a large area, such as a lobby. The triage officer, usually an emergency care physician, directs triage activity. Simplified methods of patient identification and record keeping are used to minimize the time required for paperwork. Usually, patients are assigned numbers, which are written on tags and attached to their wrists or ankles. These numbers are used to identify the radiographs and any required records.

CONCLUSION

Since one of the functions of a modern hospital is to provide care in acute situations, radiographers must expect to use the knowledge contained in this chapter on a daily basis. You should be prepared to recognize and respond appropriately to any acute condition or sudden change in a patient's status, from a simple nosebleed or wave of nausea to a major motor seizure or cardiac arrest. Remember that you are part of a team. Hospital procedures provide for the expert assistance of physicians, nurses, and code teams, so that you need not cope with crisis alone.

Study questions

1. A motor vehicle accident has brought three victims through the emergency room, and all three need radiographs. Dave Black has abrasions and pain in his right leg. Paul White has displacement of his left shoulder. The driver of the car, Mary Green, has no visible injuries but has become increasingly cross and drowsy. Which patient would cause you the most concern? What would you do?
2. What signs might alert you that a patient was experiencing airway obstruction and needed a Heimlich maneuver? Would you give CPR?
3. Mrs. Dober appears to be going into shock. What types of shock could you identify immediately? How would your treatment differ for each type?
4. Suppose it has been necessary to "call a code" in the radiology department, and the patient has been successfully resuscitated. What tasks remain to be completed before and after the patient leaves the department?

Preparation and Examination of the Gastrointestinal Tract

Vocabulary list

1. cathartic	11. irrigation
2. catheter	12. mucosa
3. colostomy	13. peristalsis
4. commode	14. pylorospasm
5. congenital	15. sigmoidoscopy
6. diverticulum	16. solution
7. fluoroscopy	17. spasm
8. hemorrhoids	18. suppository
9. Hirschsprung's disease	19. suspension
10. hygroscopic	20. viscosity

Unlike bony structures, soft tissues are frequently very difficult to demonstrate radiographically. To outline the surfaces of specific tissues, substances are used that absorb radiation to a different degree than the tissues themselves. These substances are called contrast media (*sing.,* contrast medium) and may generally be classified into four groups: barium sulfate products, aqueous iodine compounds, oily iodine compounds, and gases. This chapter focuses on the use of barium sulfate, or "barium," as a contrast medium in examination of the gastrointestinal (GI) tract. It also discusses the preparation and follow-up care for patients undergoing contrast studies of the GI tract as well as other abdominal soft tissues.

Many radiographic examinations require some type of advance preparation. One reason for preparation is to ensure that the procedure will not cause untoward side effects, as when a patient to be anesthetized fasts to avoid nausea from the anesthetic. Another reason for preparation is to cleanse the GI tract so that gas and fecal material will not obscure the structures to be demonstrated radiographically. Other preparations provide radiographic contrasts, such as tablets containing iodine compounds given to opacify the interior of the gallbladder before an oral cholecystogram examination. A specific examination may necessitate several of these steps to ensure patient comfort and safety as well as optimum visualization.

SCHEDULING AND SEQUENCING

One of the most important communications between the nursing services and radiology departments involves the scheduling of multiple diagnostic procedures that may all be ordered at one time by the referring physician. With outpatients, this communication may involve the radiology department and the nurse or receptionist in the physician's office. Consultation is often needed to decide how many procedures can be done in 1 day and to sequence them in such a way that they will not interfere with each other. For example, an upper GI series usually results in barium scattered throughout the intestinal tract for several days. Even tiny amounts of residual barium cause complications in radiographic examinations of the urinary tract and biliary system, where tiny opacifications are diagnostically significant. Residual barium in the digestive tract also causes unacceptable artifacts on abdominal computed tomography (CT) scans. For this reason, barium studies are scheduled *last* in any series of procedures.

Some departments may schedule a series of several examinations in 1 day for patients who are able to tolerate this approach. In some ways, this may be less stressful, resulting in a single bowel preparation, a single period of fasting, and perhaps a shortened hospital stay. However, the extent of examination a debilitated patient can tolerate has a limit. After one study the patient may need to rest. Also, radiologists prefer various scheduling practices. For some, it may be common procedure to schedule gallbladder and upper and lower GI studies on the same day. Others may insist on 2 to 3 days for the completion of the same examinations. Whatever the practice in your institution, it should be stated in the procedural manual and the standing orders and should be easily available to those involved in scheduling, ordering, and planning preparation.

When fiberoptic studies, such as gastroscopy or sigmoidoscopy, are ordered in conjunction with radiographic examinations requiring barium as a contrast medium, fiberoptic studies are usually done first. This avoids the possibility of the barium interfering with the visual assessment of the fiberoptic examination. Patients undergoing a gastroscopy should be NPO (nothing by mouth) for 12 hours preceding the examination. They usually receive sedation and a muscle relaxant before the physician inserts the gastroscope. If an upper GI series is to follow, one must allow sufficient time for the patient to become alert and responsive before administering the oral barium.

Another study to be considered in avoiding problems with scheduling and sequencing is the thyroid assessment test, which involves iodine uptake. The administration of contrast media containing iodine causes inaccurate results in such tests for at least 3 weeks after the radiographic study. Therefore, thyroid assessment tests must be performed before any iodinated contrast medium is administered. The following is a guide to sequencing multiple diagnostic studies for patients undergoing a comprehensive workup.

▶ Guide to sequencing order for diagnostic studies

1. All radiographic examinations *not* requiring contrast media
2. Laboratory studies for iodine uptake
3. Radiographic examinations of the urinary tract
4. Radiographic examinations of the biliary system
5. Lower GI series (barium enema)
6. Upper GI series

Two other points should be emphasized:
1. CT studies requiring intravenous (IV) contrast may be done any time after iodine uptake studies have been completed. CT studies of the abdomen or pelvis should precede examinations involving barium.
2. When scheduling multiple studies involving IV administration of iodine contrast, care must be taken that the total maximum dosages of iodine are not exceeded.

An additional consideration in patient scheduling involves deciding which patients should be scheduled first in the morning and which should be scheduled later in the day. Radiology departments always begin the daily routine with patients who must fast in preparation for examination so that they will not have to go without food for too long. If several fasting patients are scheduled, however, it must be decided which patients should be examined first. After emergency patients have been scheduled, the next priority should be pediatric and geriatric patients, since they have the most difficulty being NPO for long periods, and this may actually interfere with their recovery.

Diabetic patients who must postpone their insulin until their morning meal are also high-priority cases. Diabetic outpatients should be reminded to postpone their morning insulin until the examination is complete, even if they have been scheduled for an early appointment. If an emergency causes a delay, the patient who has had insulin may have a reaction (see Chapter 7).

PREPARATION FOR EXAMINATION

The most common and most extensive radiographic preparation is for cleansing purposes. Specific preparations vary among institutions and radiologists, and the radiographer is again referred to the procedures at the institution. Certain examinations, however, almost invariably require cleansing preparation, the primary one being the barium enema, or lower GI study. For this examination, the inner lining of the large intestine must be clean and free of all fecal matter. It is a complex undertaking to clean all the little crevices of the bowel and usually requires several steps in preparation. These may include diet, cathartics, suppositories, or enemas, and the process often consists of several or all of these methods. Once mastered, these techniques may be applied to preparations for other examinations as well.

Diet

An examination scheduled well in advance offers the opportunity to employ diet as an effective preparation. Patients may be placed on a *low-residue* diet for several days preceding the examination. At the same time, liquid intake, particularly water, is encouraged or forced, which results in rapid transit of waste through the digestive tract and less residue in the bowel. For the 24 hours immediately before the examination, the patient's diet may be restricted to *clear liquids*. These are foods that are entirely absorbed through the intestinal wall, leaving no residue. A clear liquid diet may consist of consommé or bouillon, apple juice, gelatin, and tea. Some soft drinks may also be taken. A good rule to follow is to avoid any food or drink that is not transparent. Milk products are definitely to be avoided.

Fasting is another dietary regimen that may be used in patient preparation for radiographic examinations. The NPO order is usually instituted for a limited period, approximately 8 to 12 hours, before the procedure. This ensures that the stomach will be empty at the time of examination, which is important for two reasons:

1. If the stomach is to be examined, it must be empty and "clean" so that it will produce an accurate radiographic image of its inner surfaces.
2. If the examination might cause nausea, as many IV contrast agents do occasionally, the patient is less likely to vomit. Fasting decreases the possibility that vomitus may be aspirated.

Cathartics

Cathartics, or laxative preparations, are often prescribed to aid in cleansing the bowel. Research has demonstrated that increased fluid intake enhances the effectiveness of cathartics and aids in minimizing patient discomfort. For this reason, standing orders for cathartics are accompanied by a fluid intake schedule that suggests at least 8 ounces of water or clear liquid every 2 hours between noon and midnight on the day preceding the examination.

One preparation frequently used for this purpose is castor oil, a strong, very effective cathartic agent. It is usually given in dosages of 1 to 2 ounces orally. Since its heavy, oily consistency leaves an unpleasant taste and feeling in the mouth, it is often mixed or followed with orange juice or a carbonated beverage. Castor oil has such strong, thorough action that many patients have painful spasms of the bowel and irritation of the intestinal lining after its administration. The unpleasant experience of persistent diarrhea often lasts through the night, preventing sleep. Although relatively strong patients find this preparation uncomfortable and inconvenient, its effectiveness in cleansing the bowel usually outweighs these relatively minor considerations. However, caution must be exercised in implementing castor oil preparation for elderly or frail patients who are likely to be adversely affected. When decreasing the routine strength or amount of cathartics, use of a low-residue diet and increased fluid intake become critically important to the success of the preparation.

Cathartic preparations, such as bisacodyl (Dulcolax) and citrate of magnesia, may be used instead of castor oil. One of these drugs may be the routine cathartic specified in the standing orders or may be identified as a substitute when castor oil is contraindicated. Preparations containing bismuth are contraindicated because their radiopacity causes visible "shadows" radiographically. Although a usual dosage of a specific cathartic should be stated in the procedural manual and in the standing orders, a degree of flexibility in this regard is essential. In addition to providing a gentler alternative for the debilitated patient, those with chronic or acute diarrhea may require a lower dosage or less active preparation than is usually given. On the other hand, a more active drug or a higher dose may be required for those patients who have chronic constipation or are habituated to the use of laxatives. A brief history of the patient's bowel habits helps in assessing whether the usual preparation is appropriate. Patients should always be advised of the nature of the action expected from the cathartic when it is given.

The use of a rectal suppository is sometimes valuable as a part of the bowel-cleansing preparation. Its function is to stimulate peristaltic action in the colon, which results in evacuation of the distal portion of the lower bowel. To insert a suppository, wear disposable gloves, and insert the suppository gently into the anus with one hand while holding the buttocks apart with the other hand. Using one finger, gently push the suppository past the internal sphincter and approximately 2 to 3 inches into the rectum in a superior-posterior direction. Be certain that the suppository rests in contact with the rectal mucosa, since it will not be effective if lodged in a fecal mass. Almost immediately the patient will have an urge to defecate. If this urge is acted on too quickly, the result will be evacuation of the suppository only. Thus the patient should be encouraged to retain the suppository for at least 30 minutes before evacuation.

Enemas

Enemas are another method of bowel cleansing often used in preparation for radiographic examination. This procedure consists of filling the colon with liquid to aid in dislodging and flushing out any fecal contents remaining in the lower intestinal tract. Orders for enemas are usually carried out by the nursing service in the patient's room for an inpatient or by the patient at home for an outpatient. Occasionally, this duty is assigned to the radiographer, however, and the procedure is included here for that reason. The radiographer also must be familiar with this procedure to be able to instruct those patients who need advice on taking enemas at home. An understanding of this procedure provides a basis for mastering the technique of administering the barium enema, which is routine for every radiographer.

The liquid used for a cleansing enema may be tap water or soapsuds in water. Normal saline solution, glycerin in water, and olive oil are also used occasionally. The equipment needed consists of an enema bag or pail with attached plastic or rubber tubing, a disposable rectal catheter, and apparatus from which to suspend the enema bag. An IV pole is especially useful for suspending the bag because of its mobility and its height adjustability. If tap water is to be used, fill the container with 1000 ml of tepid (105° F) water from the tap. If soapsuds are to be used, add 30 ml of liquid Castile soap and mix well. Attach the rectal catheter to the tubing, and, holding them over the sink, open the clamp. When the tubing and catheter have filled completely with the liquid, close the clamp. Filling the tubing and catheter before administration avoids instillation of air into the colon. You also need a water-soluble gel to lubricate the catheter tip. If the patient is unable to walk to the bathroom, obtain a bedpan and toilet tissue and keep them at hand.

When you are ready, explain the procedure to the patient and give instructions for assuming the Sims' position (left anterior oblique, Fig. 8-1). Cover the patient with a bath blanket for warmth and modesty. Avoid exposing the patient more than is necessary. Hang the enema container approximately 18

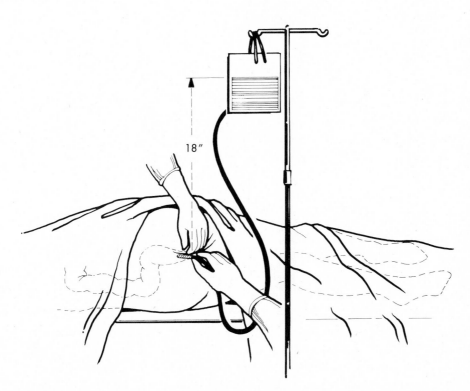

Fig. 8-1. Patient and equipment placement for enema administration.

inches above the level of the table or bed. The proper height is very important, since the position of the enema bag regulates the pressure of the liquid's flow. When the bag is too high, the increased pressure may produce a flow that is too rapid, which results in abdominal cramping. Excessive pressures may cause serious harm to patients with certain bowel conditions, such as diverticulitis.

To insert the catheter, wear disposable gloves, spread the buttocks with your fingers, and gently push the lubricated tip through the anus, directing it superiorly and anteriorly into the rectum 2 to 4 inches. At first, point the tip in the general direction of the umbilicus. If resistance is encountered, redirect the tip posteriorly to accommodate the posterior flexure of the rectum (Fig. 8-2). When inserting a rectal catheter in a female patient, take care to ensure that the catheter enters the anus and not the vagina. If you encounter any resistance to the insertion of the catheter, do *not* exert more force. Sometimes feces in the rectum may prevent proper insertion. In this case the patient may be requested to defecate before continuing with the enema. If extensive hemorrhoids (enlarged rectal veins) or other pathologic conditions interfere with catheter insertion, seek the assistance of a nurse or physician.

When the catheter is properly situated, open the clamp, allowing the liquid to flow. If the patient complains of abdominal cramping, stop the flow temporarily, and encourage the patient to relax by breathing through the mouth and panting lightly. Spasms of the bowel may occur during enema administration and often produce discomfort as well as an urge to defecate. The patient may feel "full" and believe that no further liquid can be tolerated. A spasm often occurs after the administration of about 200 ml of liquid, which is the approxi-

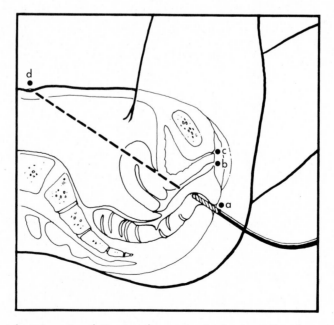

Fig. 8-2. Rectal anatomy in relation to other anatomic structures (female patient). *a,* Anus; *b,* vaginal orifice; *c,* urethral orifice; *d,* umbilicus.

mate amount required to fill the sigmoid colon. When viewing the fluoroscopic image during a barium enema examination, you will have an opportunity to observe this occurrence. If the patient has received less than 400 ml of the enema, you can be certain this feeling is caused by spasm rather than actual filling of the colon. A brief pause, perhaps with a change of position, should relieve the spasm and allow the procedure to continue. When the bag is empty, or if the patient complains of fullness after the administration of at least 750 ml, stop the flow and remove the catheter. Encourage the patient to hold the enema for 10 minutes, if possible, before going to the bathroom.

Assist the patient to the bathroom or onto the bedpan, and allow as much privacy as is consistent with patient safety. When patients require help onto the commode, use the same face-to-face assist learned in Chapter 3 for helping patients into wheelchairs. Make certain the back of the gown is clear of the seat. As soon as safety is ensured, leave the patient alone, calling attention to the emergency call button if one is available. Check with the patient at frequent intervals. If the patient or gown has become soiled, provide a clean gown, warm wet washcloth, towel, and assistance with cleansing, if needed, before the patient leaves the bathroom. A pleasant, helpful attitude helps to reassure patients, who may feel very embarrassed about having soiled themselves.

Permit ample time for the patient to expel the enema. This is very important, since spasm of the colon may deceive the patient into thinking that evacuation is complete. If the patient has expelled only a part of the enema and is unable to expel the remainder, encourage some physical activity. The process of standing up and walking around the room for a few minutes usually results in relaxation of the spasm, allowing the patient to complete the evacuation.

Many radiologists believe that one large enema that fills the entire colon is much more effective than several small ones that fill only the sigmoid colon and are discontinued at the first sign of discomfort. However, if the order calls for "enemas until clear," the procedure is repeated until no solid material can be detected in the stool. If you are checking for this result, be certain to instruct the patient not to flush the commode.

When inspecting the stool, evidence of bleeding may be noted. A black, tarry substance is indicative of blood from the upper GI tract. Fresh, red blood may result from hemorrhoids or pathologic conditions in the colon. Report these findings immediately, and do not continue with additional enemas when there is blood in the stool, except on the direct order of a physician. Since visualization of the causative lesion may be the reason for the examination, the physician may want the preparation to be continued or perhaps modified to fit the patient's condition.

The sodium phosphate (Fleet) enema is a complete, disposable enema unit containing a salt solution that is highly efficient as an evacuant. It is effective for the distal portion of the large bowel but does not contain enough fluid to cleanse the entire colon. This enema is sometimes used as a final step in a more comprehensive regimen and is often the method of choice for impromptu use in the radiology department when the patient's prior preparation has not been adequate. Complete instructions come with the product and are easily followed by radiographers and most outpatients.

When excessive gas and feces are present, cleansing preparation may be required for examinations of the sacrum and coccyx. This application is not usually found among standing preparation orders. With increasing stress on the limitation of radiation, especially to the pelvic area, perhaps cleansing before sacrum and coccyx radiography deserves to be reconsidered. A Fleet enema for this purpose is inexpensive, easy to give, and relatively tolerable for the patient. It may decrease the number of repeat exposures while increasing diagnostic accuracy.

CONTRAST MEDIA FOR GASTROINTESTINAL EXAMINATIONS

Barium sulfate

Barium sulfate is an inert inorganic salt of the chemical element barium. In the jargon of radiology, barium sulfate is typically referred to simply as "barium." It is used exclusively for radiography of the GI tract and is administered either orally or rectally. Barium is packaged in many forms, ranging from 100-pound drums of plain barium sulfate to premeasured packets containing a finely pulverized form of the medium combined with artificial flavoring and coloring. The dry powder is mixed with water just before use, forming a suspension that may be thick or thin, depending on the proportions of barium and water.

The barium itself has no flavor, but many patients find it difficult to swallow because of its chalky consistency. For oral administration, it is most palatable when thoroughly mixed with very cold water and offered with a drinking straw, which helps prevent it from coating the mouth.

For rectal administration (barium enema), the barium is mixed with tepid water (102° to 105° F) just before administration. Disposable barium enema kits are available, which include a plastic bag containing premeasured barium, enema tubing, and a rectal catheter (Fig. 8-3). When using these kits, the radiographer must simply add tepid water and shake vigorously. The bags are usually printed with graduated markings to aid in measuring the water as it is added. A bead may be situated at the junction of the bag and the tubing to prevent premature emptying of the bag. After the barium is mixed in the bag, a squeeze at the junction will dislodge the bead, allowing the tubing to fill. If the unit uses a clamp rather than a bead to prevent flow through the tubing, close the clamp while filling the bag and open it briefly to allow the tubing to fill.

The proper viscosity of the barium is important to the success of GI examinations. Usually, studies of the esophagus require a thick mixture, whereas barium enemas demand a thin one. Radiologists' preferences vary regarding the proportions to be used in regulating viscosity. This can usually be controlled with sufficient accuracy by establishing standard measurements for the amounts of barium and water to be combined for each study.

Since barium sulfate is an inert compound, it does not react chemically with the body to any appreciable extent. Allergies are almost never a problem, and few side effects occur. The principal problem complicating the use of barium is its *hygroscopic* nature, that is, its tendency to absorb water. When mixed with water, it slowly absorbs the liquid and tends to solidify in the same manner as plaster of Paris, although to a lesser degree. This problem is increased by the nor-

Fig. 8-3.

Barium enema preparation.

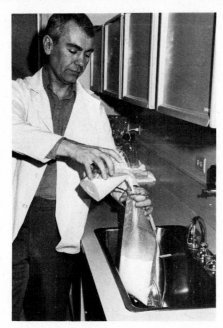

Fill enema bag with barium mixture.

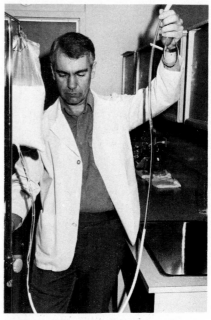

Squeeze bead or release valve at base of bag, allowing barium mixture to fill tubing.

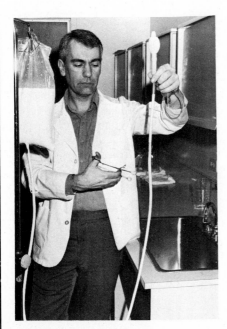

Clamp off tubing with hemostat or tube clamp. Note disposable retention catheter in this system.

mal function of the colon, which is to absorb water from the bowel contents. Care must be taken that patients with restricted bowel action do not develop a bowel obstruction as a result of barium impaction. Geriatric patients who are inactive are most prone to this problem. Therefore, increased fluids and a laxative or cathartic preparation are usually prescribed following barium studies of either the upper or lower GI tract.

Reports of allergic reactions to latex (rubber) products, including a few severe anaphylactic responses to latex enema tips, have recently increased. Some new products are being introduced that do not contain latex, but at this writing they are quite expensive and are not in general use. These new products may replace latex enema tips or may be used selectively for allergenic patients. For this reason, it may become routine to take a patient's allergy history before barium enema studies (see Chapter 9).

Iodinated media

Special aqueous iodine compounds, such as Gastrografin and Hypaque Sodium Oral, are available for contrast examination of the GI tract. These media are used only in special cases when the administration of barium sulfate might prove hazardous to the patient. They are especially useful when a rupture of the GI tract is suspected, such as perforated ulcer or ruptured appendix, because these compounds can be absorbed by the body from within the peritoneal cavity. Barium sulfate leakage into the peritoneal cavity cannot be absorbed and therefore presents a much more serious complication. The iodinated media are also used when there is high risk of barium impaction, and they are often selected for studies of neonates. Compared with barium, iodinated media are more expensive and generally produce less contrast. Also, iodinated media are not without risk. They sometimes cause serious dehydration and are hazardous if aspirated. The radiologist chooses which medium to use.

Air contrast

Barium and iodine compounds provide *positive* contrast; that is, they absorb more radiation than surrounding tissues and make a white or light shadow on the radiograph. Air and gases, on the other hand, absorb less radiation and produce *negative* contrast, or dark shadows on the film. When used in combination for double-contrast GI examinations, the barium coats the mucosal lining of the alimentary canal while the air fills the lumen. The result is a high degree of contrast, which tends to enhance the visualization of the GI mucosa.

EXAMINATIONS OF LOWER GASTROINTESTINAL TRACT
Routine barium enema

A preliminary radiograph of the abdomen may be taken before the instillation of barium. This "scout film" has diagnostic value from the radiologist's viewpoint and provides technical assistance to the radiographer. In addition, it provides a further opportunity to assess the efficacy of the preparation. If fecal material is seen in the colon on this radiograph, further preparation may be required for an optimum examination.

The administration of the barium enema is very similar to the procedure for the cleansing enema, with several significant exceptions:

1. A larger amount of liquid is prepared for a barium enema than for a cleansing enema, usually 1200 to 1500 ml.
2. The enema bag is suspended a greater distance above the table, usually 24 to 30 inches. This is necessary because the greater viscosity of the barium suspension requires greater hydrostatic pressure to maintain an adequate flow rate.
3. A larger rectal catheter is used. This may be a disposable plastic rectal tube or a retention catheter with an inflatable cuff. Disposable retention catheters are also available and are often used. The retention catheter assists the patient to retain the barium for the duration of the study.

Some radiology departments use retention catheters for all patients. In other facilities the radiographer must decide when a retention catheter is required. Patients who are alert, competent, and cooperative may be more comfortable with a plain enema tip. Others may feel more secure with a retention cuff in place. The patient's expectation regarding enema retention may be a useful guide to the radiographer in deciding which tip to use. The cuff of the retention catheter is inflated with an air pump similar to the one used with a sphygmomanometer. About 90 to 100 ml of air (one or two squeezes of the bulb) is sufficient. Some disposable enema units include a small, disposable inflation pump. Follow the directions provided with the unit.

After the tip is inserted, the patient is placed in the supine position in readiness for the fluoroscopic study. The radiologist will indicate when to start and stop the barium flow. After fluoroscopy, routine radiographs are taken (Fig. 8-4).

When the study is complete, the tube may be removed and the patient escorted to the bathroom. If a retention catheter is used, be certain to deflate the cuff before attempting to remove the catheter. In some cases it may be beneficial to place the bag below the level of the table and allow part of the barium to drain back into the bag before removing the catheter.

Most barium enema examinations include one or more postevacuation radiographs (Fig. 8-5). The best result is obtained when the patient has evacuated the barium as completely as possible. As with the cleansing enema, allow ample time for evacuation and encourage physical activity if appropriate.

Patients with unusual conditions may require special care by the radiographer when undergoing a barium enema examination. One example is the infant or child who has congenital megacolon, or Hirschsprung's disease. This condition involves a segment of distal colon in which no peristalsis occurs because of a neurologic deficiency. This causes chronic constipation and resulting enlargement of the colon to an extreme degree (Fig. 8-6).

Barium enema studies are important to the diagnosis and evaluation of this condition but may also prove hazardous. The increased area of the colon's mucosal lining provides greater opportunity for rapid, excessive absorption of water from the barium suspension. This predisposes these patients to barium impactions. Even more threatening, however, is the possibility of massive change in the fluid concentration in the blood (fluid overload). This may contribute to

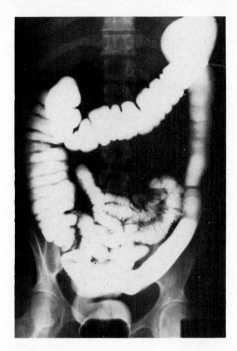

Fig. 8-4. Barium enema study demonstrates lumen of colon (anteroposterior projection). *(From Ballinger P:* Merrill's atlas of radiographic positioning and radiologic procedures, *ed 7, St Louis, 1991, Mosby–Year Book.)*

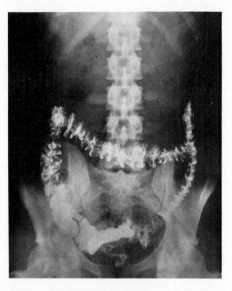

Fig. 8-5. Postevacuation radiograph demonstrates mucosal pattern of colon (posteroanterior projection). *(From Ballinger P:* Merrill's atlas of radiographic positioning and radiologic procedures, *ed 7, St Louis, 1991, Mosby–Year Book.)*

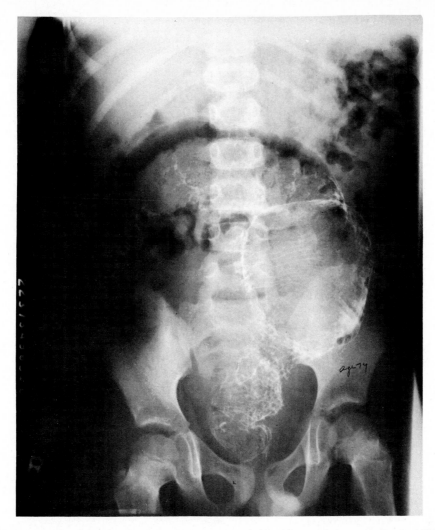

Fig. 8-6. Barium enema study (postevacuation): child with Hirschsprung's disease. *(Courtesy Harvey Tracy, Swedish Hospital, Seattle.)*

cardiac insufficiency and electrolyte imbalance. Extreme fluid overload may result in physical collapse and pulmonary edema. These hazards are minimized by mixing the barium with normal saline solution instead of tap water. Normal saline is a solution of 0.85% sodium chloride (table salt) in water and is prepared by dissolving two level teaspoons of salt in 1000 ml of tepid water.

Another situation requiring special knowledge and skill in the performance of a barium enema involves patients with colostomies. These patients have undergone surgical resections of the colon. The distal end of the remaining colon terminates in an artificial opening, called a *stoma*, in the abdominal wall. Since the patient has no voluntary control over the stoma, fecal matter is expelled through this opening automatically. These patients must wear a colostomy bag, a receptacle that fits over the opening and is sealed to the skin surrounding it. Patients with colostomies may be quite sensitive about this condition, and one must avoid any display of disgust or revulsion while caring for them. Until the procedure is sufficiently familiar to instill confidence, the student should observe an experienced radiographer.

Patients who have had a colostomy for any length of time are accustomed to performing their own colostomy care and are often most comfortable when they are allowed to empty their colostomy bag and cleanse the area themselves. Many colostomy patients irrigate their stoma daily to initiate a bowel movement at a convenient time. This allows them to wear a smaller bag or simply a protective cover. If a cleansing enema is necessary, the competent colostomy patient may do a much more effective job than the radiographer.

A special catheter is needed for the barium enema. A urinary retention (Foley) catheter may be used, since it is smaller than a rectal catheter and has a small inflatable cuff to hold it securely in place. Wear disposable gloves. With the patient in the supine position, after the colostomy bag has been removed and the area cleansed, lubricate and insert the catheter tip into the colostomy opening approximately 4 to 6 inches (Fig. 8-7). Insert the catheter gently, and do not force it if you encounter any resistance. When the catheter is properly situated, use a syringe to inflate the catheter cuff, and hold it snugly in place. Five to 10 ml of air is usually sufficient; be careful not to overinflate the cuff. Special enema catheters for colostomies are commercially available and may be used instead of the Foley catheter. Follow the manufacturer's directions.

From 500 to 700 ml of barium is usually adequate for a colostomy enema. It is instilled under fluoroscopic control under the radiologist's direction.

When the examination is complete, drain as much barium as possible back into the enema bag, deflate the catheter cuff, and remove the catheter. Provide the patient with an emesis basin or colostomy bag in which to empty the bar-

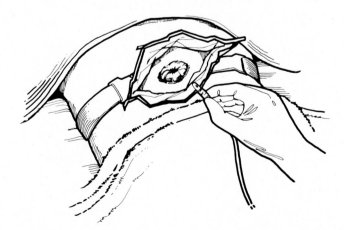

Fig. 8-7. Barium enema for patient with colostomy. Foley catheter may be used to instill barium via the stoma.

ium. The patient then requires the necessary supplies to cleanse the area and apply a fresh colostomy bag. Instructions should be given in advance to outpatients so that the necessary supplies can be brought from home to replace the colostomy bag after the examination.

Occasionally, the distal portion of the remaining colon of the colostomy patient may be studied. For this portion of the examination, the procedure is the same as for any routine barium enema, except that much less barium is needed. It may also be necessary to irrigate the distal colon to remove the barium after the study, since this part of the colon is no longer active in the elimination process.

Double-contrast barium enema

Some radiologists prefer the enhanced visualization of the mucosal lining provided by double-contrast studies for some or all of the colon examinations they perform (Fig. 8-8). A special barium mixture may be purchased for this purpose, or a preparation is thoroughly mixed to provide a suspension that is very smooth and somewhat thicker than for single-contrast studies. After the colon is filled, examined, and completely or partially evacuated, air is instilled via the enema tip using a special insufflation device or an air pump, such as the bulb used with a sphygmomanometer. Air must be instilled slowly to avoid cramping and patient discomfort. After the study the patient returns to the bathroom to evacuate the air and any residual barium.

Disposable double-contrast enema kits are available commercially. After rou-

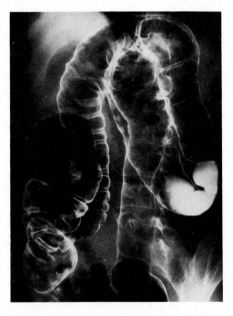

Fig. 8-8. Double-contrast barium enema enhances visualization of mucosal pattern (oblique projection). *(From Ballinger P: Merrill's atlas of radiographic positioning and radiologic procedures, ed 7, St Louis, 1991, Mosby–Year Book.)*

tine instillation of barium, these kits allow barium to be siphoned back into the bag by lowering the bag below the height of the table. Thus evacuation is accomplished without removing the patient from the fluoroscopic table. Air retained in the bag may then be instilled into the colon by turning the bag upside down and squeezing it gently. Some kits are supplied with a special enema tip that has a double lumen, allowing separate passages for air and barium and providing better control of air instillation.

UPPER GASTROINTESTINAL STUDIES

Routine upper gastrointestinal series

An upper GI series is a fluoroscopic and radiographic examination of the esophagus, stomach, and duodenum. Barium is the contrast medium for this study also and is administered orally.

Patient preparation is usually quite simple, consisting of an NPO order for approximately 8 hours before the examination. Some radiologists prefer patients not smoke on arising until after the examination, since smoking may increase gastric secretions, resulting in liquid dilution of the contrast medium in the stomach. Chewing gum is avoided for the same reason. Fig. 8-9 demonstrates the importance of adequate preparation for an upper GI study.

The patient care role of the radiographer in this examination consists of giving preliminary explanations and instructions, handing the patient the cup of barium, receiving the cup when the patient has finished it, and assisting the patient to assume various positions as directed by the radiologist. Occasionally the examination is delayed when the barium in the stomach does not empty into the duodenum because of pylorospasm. In this event, it is helpful to place the patient in the right anterior oblique position, which allows gravity to assist the normal flow of gastric contents.

Double-contrast upper gastrointestinal study

Double-contrast examination is a more recent development in upper GI studies. It enhances visualization of the mucosal surface and involves several variations in procedure (Fig. 8-10). At the beginning of the study the patient is given a gas-producing substance in the form of a tablet, powder, or carbonated beverage. This is followed by a small amount of a relatively thick barium mixture. In the recumbent position the patient is turned into various positions to ensure adequate coating of the gastric mucosa. The patient may feel the need to belch but should not do so, since the gas must be retained in the stomach to provide radiographic contrast. An anticholinergic drug, such as Glucagon, may be prescribed before examination to induce relaxation of the stomach and duodenum for better visualization.

Hypotonic duodenography

This examination is useful for the detection of lesions in the duodenum distal to the duodenal bulb and for the diagnosis of pancreatic disease. It involves the passing of a tube through the mouth or nose and into the duodenum after the administration of drugs to relax the GI tract and halt peristalsis. Barium and air

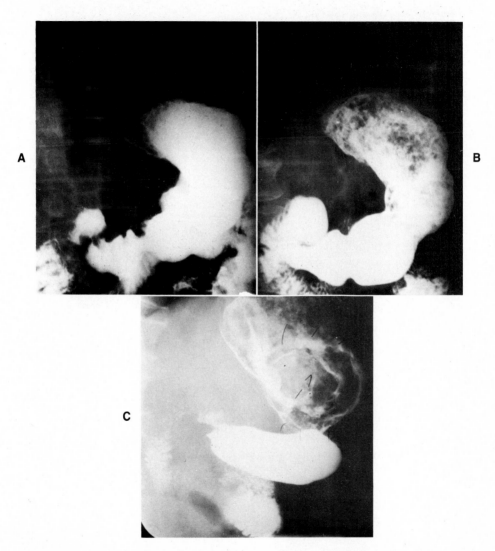

Fig. 8-9. **A,** Normal radiograph of stomach. **B,** Upper gastrointestinal study with food in stomach. **C,** Cancer of stomach. Note similarity in appearance of **B** and **C.** *(Courtesy Harvey Tracy, Swedish Hospital, Seattle.)*

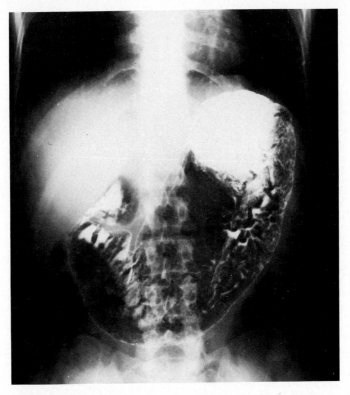

Fig. 8-10. Double-contrast upper gastrointestinal study. *(From Ballinger P: Merrill's atlas of radiographic positioning and radiologic procedures, ed 7, St Louis, 1991, Mosby—Year Book.)*

are injected through the tube via syringe to provide radiographic contrast. The use of this study is declining; it is being replaced by ultrasound, double-contrast upper GI examinations for duodenal visualization, and CT or needle biopsy for pancreatic evaluation.

FOLLOW-UP CARE

As mentioned earlier, bowel care is very important after all barium studies because of the tendency of barium to clump and harden in the bowel. This may cause constipation and, in severe cases, bowel obstruction. Prevention is far superior to the most valiant efforts at dealing with the problem. A common practice is to administer a cathartic preparation immediately after the examination. This may be a liquid, such as milk of magnesia or citrate of magnesia, or it may be a tablet, such as bisacodyl. For inpatients, this is often given by the nursing service when the patient returns to the floor. For outpatients, the cathartic may be administered by the radiographer on completion of the examination, or the patient may simply be instructed to take a laxative on returning home.

If the department's policy is merely to prescribe a laxative and leave its procurement and administration to the patient, the radiographer is responsible for being very specific in explaining the rationale for this instruction. Otherwise, the patient who has just undergone a major catharsis in preparation for the examination may not feel inclined to follow the advice and may not follow through as directed. In some hospitals it has been found that the most effective method of ensuring proper implementation of this routine is for the radiographer to administer the cathartic to *every* patient on completion of the examination. If this is your responsibility, use the method of administration of oral medication described in Chapter 6. Do not forget to chart the medication for hospital patients.

ENSURING COMPLIANCE WITH PREPARATION ORDERS

For inpatients, the nursing service is primarily responsible for performing patient preparation. The radiographer, however, has the duty to ensure that standing orders for preparations are current and to check with the patient as well as the chart to ensure that the orders have been carried out before the examination.

As previously mentioned, scout films may also be taken to evaluate patient preparation. Caution at this point may avoid the needless repetition of an examination because of inadequate preparation. Unnecessary repeat studies waste time, money, and energy in the radiology department and result in additional radiation and inconvenience to the patient. If the patient is to maintain confidence in the care received, such repetitions should be avoided.

Although the radiologist establishes the procedures, the chief radiographer usually ensures that orders are distributed and followed properly. A representative of the radiology department should meet regularly with the nursing staff to clarify any questions regarding preparations and to provide rationale. Radiographers tend to assume that "nurses know all about these things," when preparation for radiography actually is not a significant part of their education. The rationale for the examination as well as the particulars of preparation must frequently be learned on the job. Person-to-person follow-up is especially important whenever a standard procedure has been changed by the radiologist or when the two departments have recurring problems concerning preparations.

When instructing the outpatient regarding preparation for an examination, it is most helpful to have printed instructions prepared in advance. If more than one alternative is printed on any given paper, be certain to indicate, both orally and in writing, which instructions are to be followed. Review the sheet with the patient slowly, explaining any words or procedures that may not be familiar. Have the patient explain back to you what is to be done. If the patient is too young, too ill, confused, or incapable for any reason of understanding and following the instructions, give the instructions (oral and written) to the person who will be responsible for assisting the patient. Be sure to include the telephone number of the radiology department so that the patient or the patient's family may call if any questions arise after leaving the department.

When scheduling and giving instructions over the telephone, it is especially important to have patients repeat the instructions back to you in their own words, since you have fewer clues to guide you in assessing the degree to which you have been understood. A patient may say, "Yes, yes, yes," because that is the only English word he or she knows!

CONCLUSION

Examinations of the gastrointestinal tract in the radiology suite frequently require preparation by diet, cathartics, and enemas. Barium sulfate suspensions are then prepared and administered orally or rectally for visualization. The radiographer is responsible for scheduling examinations and providing instructions for preparation and follow-up care that will best serve both the diagnostic requirements and the patient's physical needs.

Study questions

1. How do gastrointestinal studies differ from routine radiographic procedures?
2. What emotional concerns might trouble a patient who is scheduled for a barium enema?
3. How would you instruct an outpatient with a colostomy to prepare for a barium enema?
4. If a patient arrived in the radiology department without being properly prepared for an examination, how would you know? What would you do?
5. What are the advantages of scheduling several diagnostic examinations for the same patient in 1 day? What are the disadvantages? Consider physical, economic, and departmental factors.

9

Contrast Media and Special Imaging Techniques

Vocabulary list

1. aqueous
2. bile
3. bilirubin
4. BUN
5. cholecystectomy
6. CT (computed tomography)
7. cystic
8. cystogram
9. diuretic
10. fiberoptic
11. forceps
12. gantry
13. hemostat
14. hepatic
15. hypothalamus
16. intrathecal
17. manometer
18. MRI (magnetic resonance imaging)
19. non-ionic

As Chapter 8 has shown, special medications or other media may be used to enhance radiographic contrast of soft tissues. Among these are barium sulfate, air, gases, aqueous iodine compounds, and iodized oils. Chapter 8 discusses barium sulfate products and their use. This chapter focuses on procedures using contrast media other than barium. It also discusses special techniques that form the basis of imaging modalities outside the specific area of radiography.

Procedures that use contrast media require special knowledge and skill for patient preparations as well as the administration of the contrast medium. Some of these examinations are very sophisticated procedures. It is not within the scope of this book to deal with the specifics of each examination because exact techniques vary greatly among departments and radiologists. Some of these studies, however, are so integral to the radiographer's work that they are performed routinely. A more thorough understanding of them will help you form the professional judgments required for outstanding performance in these situations.

CONTRAST MEDIA

Air and gases

Air and gases are easily penetrated by x-rays and therefore appear black or very dark on a radiograph. Cavities filled with air give a clear outline of the surrounding soft tissues, which have a lighter appearance because of their greater degree of radiation absorption. In addition to double-contrast studies of the colon and stomach (see Chapter 8), air or gas is sometimes used as a contrast agent in arthrography. Gas is sometimes also used as a contrast agent in myelography for patients who are allergic to iodinated contrast media. Carbon dioxide (CO_2) has clear advantages over room air as a diagnostic gas because it is absorbed much faster by the body than the nitrogen in air. Some departments stock CO_2 in a pressurized cylinder for use in air-contrast enemas and other studies.

In the past, gas was introduced into the abdominal cavity to study the female pelvic organs (pelvic pneumonography) and into the spinal canal to delineate the ventricles of the brain (ventriculography). These procedures have now been replaced by less invasive ultrasound and computed tomography (CT) examinations.

Iodinated media

Table 9-1 lists many of the diagnostic contrast agents found in the radiology department, and Table 9-2 categorizes these media according to their applications. For more specific information regarding the content, strength, contraindications, and precautions, the radiographer is referred to the drug package inserts or the "Diagnostic Products Information" section of the *Physician's Desk Reference* (PDR).

Iodine compounds absorb radiation to a greater degree than blood or soft tissues and therefore produce a white or light shadow on the radiograph. This causes any organ or blood vessel that contains the contrast agent to stand out

Table 9-1

Iodinated contrast media for radiography

Trade name	Generic name	Iodine salts (% weight/volume)	Approved uses
Amipaque	Metrizamide	48.25	Myelography, CT (intrathecal)
Angio-Conray	Iothalamate meglumine	80	Angiography
Bilopaque	Tyropanoate sodium	57.4	Oral cholecystography
Cardiografin	Diatrizoate meglumine	85	Angiography
Cholebrine	Iocetamic acid	62	Oral cholecystography
Cholografin Meglumine	Iodipamide meglumine	52	IV cholangiography
Cholografin Meglumine for Infusion	Iodipamide meglumine	10.3	IV drip infusion cholangiography and cholecystography
Conray	Iothalamate meglumine	60	Multipurpose
Conray-30	Iothalamate meglumine	30	IV urography, CT
Conray-43	Iothalamate meglumine	43	IV urography, venography, CT, DSA
Conray-325	Iothalamate sodium	54.3	IV urography
Conray-400	Iothalamate sodium	66.8	Angiography
Cysto-Conray	Iothalamate meglumine	43	Retrograde pyelography
Cysto-Conray II	Iothalamate meglumine	17.2	Cystourethrography
Cystografin	Diatrizoate meglumine	30	Cystourethrography
Cystografin—Dilute	Diatrizoate meglumine	18	Retrograde cystourethrography
Diatrizoate Meglumine Injection 76%	Diatrizoate meglumine	76	IV urography, aortography, pediatric angiocardiography, peripheral angiography
Dionosil	Propyliodone		Bronchography
Ethiodol	Ethiodized oil		Lymphography
Gastrografin	Diatrizoate meglumine and diatrizoate sodium	76	Gastrointestinal studies, CT body scans
Hexabrix	Sodium meglumine ioxaglate	32	Angiography and multipurpose
Hypaque 76	Diatrizoate meglumine and diatrizoate sodium	76	Multipurpose
Hypaque Sodium Oral Powder and Hypaque Sodium Oral Solution	Diatrizoate sodium	59.87	Gastrointestinal studies
Hypaque Sodium 20%	Diatrizoate sodium	20	Retrograde pyelography
Hypaque Sodium 25%	Diatrizoate sodium	25	IV urography, CT
Hypaque Sodium 50%	Diatrizoate sodium	50	Multipurpose
Hypaque Meglumine 30%	Diatrizoate meglumine	30	IV urography, CT
Hypaque Meglumine 60%	Diatrizoate meglumine	60	Multipurpose
Hypaque-Cysto	Diatrizoate meglumine	30	Cystourethrography
Hypaque-M 90%	Diatrizoate meglumine and diatrizoate sodium	90	Angiocardiography, aortography, angiography, urography, hysterosalpingography
Isopaque 280	Meglumine metrizoate	60	Multipurpose

IV, Intravenous; *CT*, computed tomography; *DSA*, digital subtraction angiography. Continued.

Table 9-1

Iodinated contrast media for radiography—cont'd

Trade name	Generic name	Iodine salts (% weight/volume)	Approved uses
Isopaque 440	Meglumine metrizoate	82	Angiography
Isovue-128	Iopamidol	12.8	Arterial DSA
Isovue-200	Iopamidol	41	Peripheral venography
Isovue-300	Iopamidol	30	Peripheral arteriography
Isovue-370	Iopamidol	37	Selective visceral arteriography
Isovue-M 200	Iopamidol	41	Thoracic myelography
Isovue-M 300	Iopamidol	61	Total column myelography
MD-76	Diatrizoate meglumine and diatrizoate sodium	76	IV urography, angiography, CT
MD-Gastroview	Diatrizoate meglumine and diatrizoate sodium		Gastrointestinal studies, CT body scans
Omnipaque 140	Iohexol	*	Arterial DSA
Omnipaque 180	Iohexol	*	Myelography
Omnipaque 240	Iohexol	*	Multipurpose
Omnipaque 300	Iohexol	*	Arteriography, Aortography, CT (IV and intrathecal)
Omnipaque 350	Iohexol	*	Aortography, angiocardiography, CT (IV), IV DSA
Optiray 160	Ioversol	34	Arterial DSA
Optiray 240	Ioversol	51	Cerebral angiography, venography
Optiray 320	Ioversol	68	Angiography, IV urography, CT
Optiray 350	Ioversol	74	Coronary arteriography, left ventriculography
Oragrafin Calcium (granules)	Ipodate calcium	61.7	Cholecystography
Oragrafin Sodium (capsules)	Ipodate sodium	61.4	Cholecystography
Pantopaque	Iophendylate		Myelography
Renografin-60	Diatrizoate meglumine and diatrizoate sodium	60	Multipurpose
Renografin-76	Diatrizoate meglumine and diatrizoate sodium	76	Multipurpose
Reno-M-30	Diatrizoate meglumine	30	Retrograde pyelography
Reno-M-60	Diatrizoate meglumine	60	Multipurpose
Reno-M-Dip	Diatrizoate meglumine	30	Urography infusion, CT venography
Renovist	Diatrizoate meglumine and diatrizoate sodium	69.3	Multipurpose
Renovist II	Diatrizoate meglumine and diatrizoate sodium	57.6	Multipurpose
Renovue-65	Iodamide meglumine	65	IV urography
Renovue-Dip	Iodamide meglumine	24	Urography infusion

*Iohexol contains 46.38% iodine. The numerical designations for Omnipaque indicate mg/ml of iohexol in solution.

(**Table 9-1**)——————————————————————————————————————
Iodinated contrast media for radiography—cont'd

Trade name	Generic name	Iodine salts (% weight/volume)	Approved uses
Sinografin	Diatrizoate meglumine and iodipamide meglumine	82.5	Hysterosalpingography
Skiodan	Methiodal sodium	20, 40	Retrograde pyelography
Telepaque	Iopanoic acid	66.7	Oral cholecystography
Vascoray	Iothalamate meglumine and iothalamate sodium	78	Angiography

from the surrounding tissues, which appear darker. Thus many different structures can be defined more sharply than would be possible without contrast media.

Iodized oils.   Iodized oils are specialized contrast agents that were developed for studies in which absorption of contrast into the surrounding tissues or mixing of contrast with body fluids was undesired. The principal use of iodized oil today is for lymphangiography; the agent used is Ethiodol. Iodized oils were once frequently used for hysterosalpingography (examination of the fallopian tubes), bronchography, myelography, and delineation of fistulous tracts caused by infection. These applications are now quite rare or obsolete, with iodized oils replaced almost entirely by low-osmolar aqueous contrast agents.

Aqueous iodine compounds.   Aqueous iodine compounds are by far the most frequently used contrast agents other than barium. These media are stocked in the radiology department in a wide variety of types, sizes, and strengths. Although some of these products are approved for one specific purpose, others have broader application. These multipurpose agents may be used for urography or angiography, or they may be injected directly into the structures to be visualized, such as the common bile duct for cholangiography or the joint capsule in arthrography. When injected intravascularly, they circulate in the blood and are excreted by the kidneys. When injected into other structures, they are reabsorbed into the bloodstream and then excreted via the urinary tract.

Two common, versatile compounds are diatrizoate meglumine and diatrizoate sodium. Each chemical has individual properties that are desired. The sodium salts are made up of relatively small molecules and contain more iodine per molecule, so that in equal concentrations they are more radiopaque than their meglumine counterparts. Meglumine (methylglucamine) salts are somewhat less toxic and are more soluble in water. Some contrast agents, such as Renografin 60 and Hypaque 76, include both chemicals. These agents are referred to as *high-osmolar contrast agents* (HOCAs) because of their relatively high osmolality compared with the newer generation of aqueous iodine contrast media.

Table 9-2

Radiographic studies using iodinated contrast media

Examination	Structures visualized	Route of administration	Examples of contrast media used
Angiography			
Aortography	Abdominal or thoracic aorta	Arterial catheter	Conray-400, Hypaque-M 90%, Isopaque 440, Renografin-76,
Angiocardiography	Heart and surrounding great vessels	Arterial catheter	Vascoray, Omnipaque 300, Omnipaque 350,
Digital Subtraction angiography (DSA)	Cerebral vasculature, aorta and branches	Arterial catheter	Isovue-128, Optiray 160
		IV catheter	Omnipaque 350
Peripheral arteriography	Arteries of the extremities	Arterial catheter or percutaneous injection	Hypaque Meglumine 60%, Renografin-60,
Peripheral venography	Veins of the extremities	Percutaneous, IV injection	Conray, Reno-M-60, Renovist, Omnipaque 300,
Cerebral angiography	Cerebral vasculature	Arterial catheter or percutaneous injection	Isovue-300, Isovue-370, Hexabrix, Niopam
Selective visceral arteriography	Renal, celiac, splenic, or coronary arteries, for example	Arterial catheter	Hypaque 76, Renografin-76, Vasocoray, Omnipaque 300, Isovue-300, Isovue-370, Hexabrix, Niopam
Splenoportography	Splenic artery and portal system	Percutaneous injection	Hypaque Meglumine 60%, Hypaque Sodium 50%, Renografin-60, Hexabrix
Biliary system			
Cholecystography	Gallbladder	Oral	Bilopaque, Cholebrine, Oragrafin (Calcium or Sodium), Telepaque
Cholangiography	Hepatic, cystic, and common bile ducts	Oral	
		IV	Cholografin Meglumine, Biligram
		Operative T tube Percutaneous	Hypaque Meglumine 60%, Hypaque Sodium 50%, Renografin-60, Reno-M-60
Endoscopic retrograde cholangiopancreatography (ERCP)	Common bile and pancreatic ducts	Catheterization via gastroscope	Omnipaque 240

Table 9-2

Radiographic studies using iodinated contrast media—cont'd

Examination	Structures visualized	Route of administration	Examples of contrast media used
Spinal studies			
Myelography	Spinal canal (sub-arachnoid space)	Lumbar puncture	Amipaque, Isovue-M 200 and 300, Omnipaque 180
Discography	Intervertebral disc	Direct injection	Hypaque Meglumine 60%, Renografin-60
Urinary tract studies			
Urography and nephrography	Excretory study of kidneys, ureters, and bladder	IV injection	Hypaque Sodium 50%, Hypaque Meglumine 60%, Conray, Conray-325, Renografin-60, Renovue-65, Hexabrix
Retrograde pyelography	Kidney pelves, calyces, and ureters	Ureteral catheter	Cysto-Conray, Hypaque Sodium 20%, Reno-M-30
Cystourethrography	Urinary bladder, urethra	Urinary catheter	Cysto-Conray II, Cystografin, Hypaque-Cysto
Miscellaneous studies			
Arthrography	Joints (e.g., knee, shoulder, ankle)	Direct injection	Hypaque Meglumine 60%, Renografin-60, Omnipaque 240 and 300
Bronchography	Bronchial tree	Laryngeal cannula or bronchial catheter	Dionosil
Computed tomography scans	Contrast enhancement of anatomy examined	IV injection or infusion	Conray-30, Hypaque Meglumine 30%, Hypaque Sodium 25%, Omnipaque
	Spinal canal (sub-arachnoid space)	Lumbar puncture	Omnipaque 240, Isovue-M 200
Hysterosalpingography	Uterus and fallopian tubes	Cervical cannula	Sinografin, Hypaque-M 90%, Hexabrix
Lymphography	Lymph vessels and lymph nodes	Direct injection of lymphatic vessels (feet and/or hands)	Ethiodol
Magnetic resonance imaging (MRI)	Brain, spinal cord	IV injection	Magnevist, ProHance

In the 1980s a new assortment of aqueous contrast media was made available to the radiology market. These products are referred to as *low-osmolality contrast agents* (LOCAs) because of their ability to deliver a relatively high concentration of iodine with fewer particles in solution than conventional contrast media. The first of these agents was metrizamide (Amipaque), and its application was primarily centered on intrathecal (within the spinal canal) injection for myelography, even though it was also approved for intravascular injection. Newer LOCAs for multipurpose use, such as meglumine ioxaglate (Hexabrix), are now replacing metrizamide. Some LOCAs are also designated as *non-ionic* because they do not dissociate into two charged particles when placed in solution. Examples include iopamidol (Isovue, Niopam) and iohexol (Omnipaque). These agents are less toxic than conventional contrast media and are less likely to stimulate an anaphylactic response. They are also more comfortable for the patient, producing less heat and discomfort when injected.

The desired features of these new products are considerably offset by their cost, which may be 6 to 18 times that of their conventional counterparts. With increased emphasis on cost containment in health care and restrictions by third-party payers on the amounts allowable for diagnostic procedures, the decision of which medium to use is difficult. Most radiology departments are now using LOCAs for certain procedures and for all patients whose allergy history or physical condition places them at greater risk.

Risk factors that may influence the choice or dosage of media include any history of compromised renal, cardiac, or respiratory function and any history of prior allergies. The weight given to various risk factors varies with the institution and physicians involved. As of this writing, many departments are still struggling to balance the risks, liabilities, and costs involved as they formulate the policies that will determine which media will be used in the future.

Many different concentrations of contrast agents are available for various applications. Generally a higher concentration produces a greater degree of contrast visualization and is desired when significant dilution of the medium by blood or urine is anticipated. Greater concentrations also have a greater viscosity, which is an important consideration in calculating flow rate, injection time, and needle size. Remember that concentration usually affects toxicity, with higher concentrations tending to be more toxic.

When used intravenously, these agents may be injected directly using a syringe and intravenous (IV) catheter, or butterfly set, or they may be administered in a diluted form through an IV drip infusion. Either method, or both, may be employed for contrast enhancement when doing CT scans.

Toxic and allergic responses.   Procedures involving IV or intrathecal administration of iodine contrast are not without risk. An informed consent may be required, and a careful history is essential. Patients may have allergic reactions because of sensitivity to iodine or some other component of the contrast medium. Toxic responses may result from poor kidney function or an overdose of the contrast agent.

Renal failure or compromised renal function impairs the patient's ability to eliminate the contrast and may result in a toxic response. Therefore you should check the blood chemistry section of inpatient charts to ensure that the blood urea nitrogen (BUN) and creatinine levels are within normal limits, that is, BUN, 8 to 25 mg/dl, and creatinine, 0.6 to 1.5 mg/dl. Report abnormal test levels to the radiologist before the administration of iodinated contrast. With outpatients, screen for a history of kidney disease or kidney failure and report positive responses.

Since several different departments may use iodine contrast (radiography, cardiovascular laboratory, CT), the patient may be scheduled for more than one contrast examination in a limited period. For instance, a patient brought to the emergency room with abdominal pain may be suspected of having a kidney stone and sent to the radiology department for an IV urogram. If this study is negative, the patient may be admitted and transferred to the care of another physician, who orders a CT scan of the abdomen. The contrast dose for the two procedures combined may exceed the 24-hour maximum dose. One expects that records are kept, transferred with the patient, and read by those who may order additional tests. However, records are sometimes slow to follow, and it only takes a moment to ask the patient whether any other tests have been done recently.

When the history has documented the reason for the examination, the patient's renal status, and any other recent contrast studies, the next step is an allergy history.

The radiologist establishes the exact procedure for taking an allergy history. Some radiologists prefer to take the history themselves. Many institutions use a written form for this purpose (see Appendix H). The procedure usually consists of asking the patient the following questions:

1. Are you allergic to anything that you know of?
2. If so, what are you allergic to?
3. How do you react (what happens) when you contact this substance?
4. Do you ever experience hay fever, asthma, or hives?
5. If so, do you know what causes this?
6. Have you ever had a radiographic examination of the kidneys or arteries or other study involving the injection of a contrast agent?
7. If so, did you have any complications related to the drugs used?

You may need to ask additional questions to identify possible heart trouble, hypertension, and respiratory problems that may influence the choice of contrast agent or help in determining the dose.

If the patient's history suggests a high risk of allergic response, the procedure may be cancelled, or it may be preceded by the administration of an antihistamine or corticosteroid drug to minimize the possibility of reaction. A test dose of the contrast medium may be injected intravenously and the patient observed carefully for several minutes. If no symptoms are noted, the injection is then continued. The radiographer must be prepared to respond to a reaction from the test dose, since serious allergic responses have been reported in sensitive individuals with only 1 ml of the medium injected.

Severe reactions to contrast media are not common, but they do occur. Although the physician should be within the immediate area, the radiographer often notes the first signs of a reaction. Your ability to cope with such emergencies depends on your recognition of symptoms and your knowledge of the actions and treatment to follow (see Chapter 7). Emergency supplies and equipment must be readily available.

State laws or regulations may govern whether radiographers are allowed to start IV lines and perform IV injections. Institutional requirements or prohibitions may exist as well. In most situations when radiographers are permitted to administer IV contrast, some sort of certification is required. Be aware of the standards that prevail in your hospital, and keep your qualifications up to date. See Chapter 6 for IV injection procedures.

CONTRAST EXAMINATIONS OF URINARY SYSTEM

Intravenous urography

Intravenous urograms are sometimes called intravenous pyelograms, or IVPs (terminology derived from roots signifying visualization of the kidney pelvis). Since the scope of the examination usually includes the entire urinary tract, *urogram* is a more accurate term, although less often used.

The IV urogram is a functional study of the urinary system accomplished by the injection of an aqueous iodine contrast medium, such as Hypaque Meglumine 60%, Renografin-60, or Isovue-300. The contrast medium mixes and circulates with the blood until it reaches the kidneys, which extract it. As a component of urine, the contrast medium opacifies first the outer portion of the kidney as it fills the tiny vessels and glomeruli in the cortex and the collecting tubules in the medulla. This imparts a hazy opacification to the entire kidney structure, which quickly disappears with normal function. Films taken during this phase are referred to as *nephrograms* and are used especially in the evaluation of patients with hypertension.

As the contrast medium is collected, it is channeled into the calyces and pelves of the kidneys, clearly outlining these structures. As the pelves fill, the opaque urine begins to flow through the ureters and into the bladder (Fig. 9-1). Thus each portion of the urinary tract may be visualized, in turn, by the timing of the radiographic sequence.

Preparation for urography usually includes cleansing of the bowel to avoid gas and fecal shadows that could obscure structures of interest. NPO (nothing by mouth) orders are given to avoid nausea and to create a moderate degree of dehydration, resulting in a greater concentration of the contrast medium in the kidneys. Diuretic drugs should not be given for 24 hours before the examination, since they tend to dilute the contrast agent with body fluids during excretion.

In preparation for the injection, the radiographer checks the emergency supplies and equipment and sets up the IV medication tray (see Chapter 6), including the vial of contrast medium, syringe, and needle or IV catheter of the appropriate size. For drip infusion administration, you need instead a drip bottle of dilute contrast medium and an IV infusion set. Dosage varies depending on the medium used, the radiologist's preference, and the patient's weight and age. Some radiologists use 1.0 ml of contrast per pound of body weight, with a maximum limit of 100 ml. After explaining the procedure and introducing the

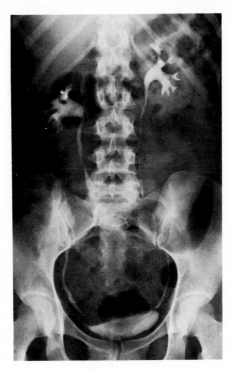

Fig. 9-1. Intravenous urogram. *(From Ballinger P:* Merrill's atlas of radiographic and radiologic procedures, *ed 7, St Louis, 1991, Mosby—Year Book.)*

patient to the radiologist, the radiographer assists with the injection, after which the radiographer proceeds with the technical aspects of the examination. The patient must be closely monitored for signs of adverse reaction to the contrast medium.

Cystography

Several other studies of the urinary tract deserve mention. The cystogram provides contrast imaging of the internal contours of the urinary bladder by means of an aqueous iodine medium injected via a urinary catheter (Fig. 9-2).

Voiding cystourethrograms (VCUGs) examine both the urinary bladder and the urethra. The bladder is filled with contrast, as for a cystogram; the catheter is removed; and fluoroscopy with spot films records the contours of the urethra and the action of the bladder as the patient voids. Some institutions have highly specialized equipment for measuring urinary force and flow rate, and these measurements may be taken in conjunction with the VCUG study.

When a cystogram is ordered, the patient is usually sent to the radiology department with a retention catheter in place. If an outpatient study is being done or if the catheter must be replaced, the hospital will have a specific standing order indicating who will insert the catheter. A nurse or orderly may be requested to come to the department for this duty, or the radiologist or urologist

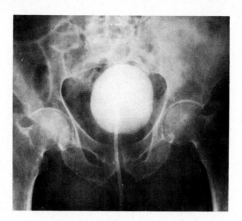

Fig. 9-2. Cystogram. *(From Ballinger P: Merrill's atlas of radiographic and radiologic procedures, ed 7, St Louis, 1991, Mosby–Year Book.)*

may catheterize the patient. In some hospitals this procedure is performed by radiographers who have been trained in catheterization technique (see pp. 223 to 226). The audiovisual or nursing education department of your college or the in-service department of your hospital will have slides, videotapes, and anatomical models, which are invaluable in learning the theory and technique of catheterization.

The chief concern in performing a cystogram is the possibility of introducing bacteria into the urinary tract, thus causing an infection in a patient who may already have a compromised urinary system. A cystogram is a minor sterile procedure that does not require gowning. When the catheter is in place, the contrast medium (Cystografin or Hypaque-Cysto) is poured into a 50 to 100 ml catheter-tip syringe and allowed to flow by gravity through the catheter and into the bladder. The radiographer's role includes explaining the procedure to the patient, assembling the necessary equipment and supplies, assisting the physician with injection, and completing the technical aspects of the procedure. In some departments, cystography may be performed solely by radiographers. When that is the case, a suggested procedure is as follows:

1. Obtain all needed equipment and position it conveniently. Place the patient on the table in the supine position and cover with a sheet, allowing access to the catheter. Explain the procedure.
2. Wash your hands. Don gloves.
3. Cleanse the catheter drainage tube junction with antiseptic if the catheter is to be left in place after the procedure.
4. Separate catheter from drainage tubing, taking care not to contaminate either end. Protect the end of the tubing with dry, sterile gauze or a sterile plastic cover. Place the tubing so it will not be contaminated. Hold the catheter in your nondominant hand.
5. Fill the syringe with contrast medium and place its tip into the end of the catheter. Hold the catheter and syringe in the vertical position to prevent air from being injected into the bladder, and allow the contrast medium

to flow into the bladder by gravity. It is not necessary to push the plunger of the syringe.

6. When all the contrast medium has run in, clamp the catheter until the radiographs have been completed.
7. Remove gloves. Wash your hands.
8. When the study is complete, wash hands, don gloves, and unclamp the catheter. Allow the contrast/urine to drain into a disposable container.
9. Cleanse the end of the catheter with antiseptic. Reconnect to drainage tubing, taking care not to contaminate the ends.
10. Remove equipment. Remove gloves and wash your hands.
11. Assist the patient from the radiographic table.
12. Charting should include the amount of urine discarded if patient is under orders to have intake and output (I & O) recorded.

Cystograms may be performed in conjunction with a cystoscopic procedure (fiberoptic study of the bladder). Under these circumstances the patient is sedated, and a surgical nurse assists the physician. The radiographer's role is almost exclusively technical.

➠ Catheterization technique

For routine cystography (both male and female), size 14 or 16 Foley (retention) catheters are recommended.

Female catheterization procedure
1. Wash hands.
2. Obtain and assemble equipment: catheter, antiseptic solution, cotton balls, lubricant, specimen bottle, waste urine receptacle, drapes, forceps, syringe, needle, sterile water, and sterile gloves. (All are commercially available in a sterile, disposable tray.)
3. Check patient identification and explain the procedure. Provide privacy.
4. Position patient supine with hips and knees flexed and legs separated, exposing perineum. Drape torso and legs.
5. Place tray between patient's legs. Open tray and don gloves, using aseptic technique (see Chapter 4).
6. Position sterile drapes by first placing a drape under the buttocks. (Cuff drape around your hands to avoid contaminating gloves.) Place the fenestrated (window) drape over the pubis and genital area, exposing the labia.
7. Pour antiseptic over cotton balls. Open lubricant and squeeze some onto the drape.
8. Using nondominant hand, separate the labia to provide a clear view of the urethral orifice (Fig. 9-3). NOTE: Left hand is now contaminated and will not be used to handle sterile objects.
9. Cleanse the genital area. Using your fingers or the small forceps, grasp an antiseptic cotton ball with the dominant hand. With a single, firm, downward stroke, cleanse the far side of the labia from pubis to anus; discard cotton ball. Repeat this step for near side of labia, and again, with a third cotton ball, down the center of the labia, directly over the urethral orifice.
10. Place the distal (wide) end of the catheter in the drainage receptacle. With

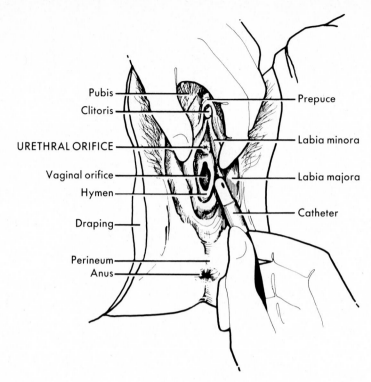

Pubis
Clitoris
URETHRAL ORIFICE
Vaginal orifice
Hymen
Draping
Perineum
Anus
Prepuce
Labia minora
Labia majora
Catheter

Fig. 9-3. Topographical anatomy of female perineum. Note location of urethral orifice.

your dominant hand or the large forceps, grasp the catheter about 3 inches from its tip. Apply lubricant to the tip.

11. Still exposing the orifice with the nondominant hand, insert the tip of the catheter gently into the orifice, guiding it posteriorly and superiorly about 2 inches. Slight resistance may be encountered at the internal urethral sphincter, which will relax when the patient exhales. Release the pressure on the catheter. If urine does not flow, the catheter tip may be lodged against the bladder wall. Rotate the catheter between thumb and forefinger, and insert up to 1 inch farther.

12. If a specimen is needed, clamp the catheter after a small amount of urine has drained into the receptacle. Transfer the distal end of the catheter into the specimen bottle. Release the forceps, allowing at least 30 ml (1 ounce) of urine to flow into the bottle. Stop the flow, and transfer the catheter end back to the drainage receptacle; unclamp. NOTE: Normally the bladder is emptied completely in preparation for the cystogram. However, no more than 1000 ml should be removed at one time, since the patient may go into shock. (Some hospitals have policies that restrict the draining of urine to fewer than 1000 ml of urine at one time. Be familiar with the institutional policies that apply.)

13. Inflate the retention balloon by using a syringe and needle to inject 5 ml of sterile water into the balloon valve on the catheter's end. (The valve is self-sealing when the needle is removed.) Tug gently on the catheter to be certain that it will be properly retained. Firm resistance indicates proper inflation of the balloon.

14. Chart the amount of urine removed if the patient is under orders for the recording of intake and output (I & O). Patient is now ready for cystography. Remove gloves and discard tray, unless a combination catheterization and cystography tray has been used. In this case, change gloves and proceed with the cystogram.
15. To remove catheter, wash hands, then deflate the retention balloon. This may be accomplished by using a scissors to snip off the balloon valve and allowing the water to drain into a basin, or by using a 10 ml syringe and needle to withdraw the water through the valve. Place paper towels under the catheter. Remove by pulling gently, and discard. Cleanse the genital area with a towel or cotton balls and attend to the patient's comfort.

Male catheterization procedure
1. Wash hands.
2. Obtain and assemble equipment: catheter, antiseptic solution, cotton balls, lubricant, specimen bottle, waste urine receptacle, drapes, forceps, syringe, needle, sterile water, and sterile gloves. (All are commercially available in a sterile, disposable tray.)
3. Check patient identification and explain the procedure. Provide privacy.
4. Place the patient in the supine position, with legs extended and relaxed. Drape the torso down to the pubis and the legs up to the groin, leaving the penis exposed.
5. Place tray adjacent to patient's hip on the side nearest you. Open tray and don gloves using aseptic technique (see Chapter 4).
6. Position sterile drapes by first placing a drape under the buttocks. (Cuff drape around your hands to avoid contaminating gloves.) Place the fenestrated (window) drape over the penis.
7. Pour antiseptic over cotton balls. Open lubricant and squeeze some onto the drape.
8. Place the penis in the palm of the nondominant hand and grasp it with the third and fourth fingers. Holding the penis in a vertical position, use the thumb and forefinger to spread the urinary orifice (Fig. 9-4). Left hand is now contaminated. NOTE: Handle the penis firmly, but not roughly. (Too gentle a touch may stimulate an erection.)
9. Using the dominant hand, pick up an antiseptic cotton ball and cleanse the penis. Use a circular motion and work toward the tip; discard cotton ball. Use a second cotton ball to cleanse firmly but gently over the orifice; discard.
10. Grasp the catheter with the large forceps about 4 inches from its tip and place the distal end in drainage receptacle. Lubricate the catheter tip.
11. Still holding the penis firmly in the nondominant hand, draw it forward and upward (60 to 90 degrees toward the legs), stretching it slightly. This action will straighten the urethra for easy insertion of the catheter. Insert the catheter gently and slowly about 7 inches. (This will require releasing your grasp on the catheter and regrasping it about 4 inches distal to the original hold.) NOTE: Resistance may be felt as the catheter passes the internal urethral sphincter. Use continuous, gentle pressure, and instruct the patient to try to void. *Do not force insertion of the catheter.* If there seems to be an obstruction or stricture, stop the procedure and call the physician.

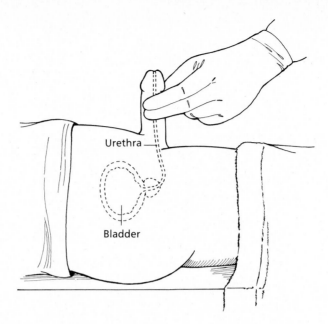

Fig. 9-4.   Position of penis for male catheterization. *(From Potter PA, Perry A: Basic nursing, ed 2, St Louis, 1991, Mosby–Year Book.)*

12. If a specimen is needed, clamp the catheter after a small amount of urine has drained into the receptacle. Transfer the distal end of the catheter into the specimen bottle. Release the forceps, allowing at least 30 ml (1 ounce) of urine to flow into the bottle. Stop the flow, and transfer the catheter end back to the drainage receptacle; unclamp. NOTE: Normally the bladder is emptied completely in preparation for the cystogram. However, no more than 1000 ml should be removed at one time, since the patient may go into shock. (Some hospitals have policies that restrict the draining of urine to fewer than 1000 ml of urine at one time. Be familiar with the institutional policies that apply.)

13. Inflate the retention balloon by using a syringe and needle to inject 5 ml of sterile water into the balloon valve on the catheter's end. (The valve is self-sealing when the needle is removed.) Tug gently on the catheter to be certain that it will be properly retained. Firm resistance indicates proper inflation of the balloon.

14. Chart the amount of urine removed if the patient is under orders for the recording of intake and output (I & O). Patient is now ready for cystography. Remove gloves and discard tray, unless a combination catheterization and cystography tray has been used. In this case, change gloves and proceed with the cystogram.

15. To remove catheter, wash hands, then deflate the retention balloon. This may be accomplished by using a scissors to snip off the balloon valve and allowing the water to drain into a basin, or by using a 10 ml syringe and needle to withdraw the water through the valve. Place paper towels under the catheter. Remove by pulling gently, and discard. Cleanse the genital area with a towel or cotton balls and attend to the patient's comfort.

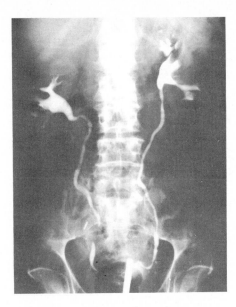

Fig. 9-5. Retrograde pyelogram.

Retrograde pyelography

Another urographic examination often performed in conjunction with cystos-
copy is the retrograde pyelogram. Under cystoscopic visualization, long, slender
catheters are inserted into the ureters, and an aqueous iodine compound, such
as Reno-M-30, is injected into the kidney pelves via the catheters. This study
provides radiographic visualization of the anatomical form of the pelves, calyces, and ureters (Fig. 9-5). The radiographer's role is almost exclusively technical.

CONTRAST EXAMINATIONS OF BILIARY SYSTEM

Oral cholecystography

The gallbladder is usually examined using an orally administered contrast medium in the form of tablets (Telepaque, Bilopaque, Oragrafin) or Oragrafin
granules. The medium is dissolved in the stomach, absorbed in the small bowel,
extracted from the blood by the liver, and used as one of the components of
bile that is then stored in the gallbladder. The tablets are most often prescribed
for routine procedures, whereas the granules provide more rapid visualization
when time is an important factor. The granules also result in increased visualization of the biliary ducts. Granules are mixed with a specified quantity of water to form a solution that the patient drinks. Tablets and granules are sometimes combined for specific studies.

Preparation for the oral cholecystogram begins early on the day preceding
the examination. For breakfast or lunch on this day, the patient's diet must include some fat. Two strips of crisp bacon or two pats of butter adequately fill
this requirement. This is especially important for patients who have been on a

low-fat diet by preference or by prescription. The gallbladder's function is to concentrate and store bile. The presence of dietary fat causes the gallbladder to contract and release bile into the duodenum to aid in the digestion of fats. If no stimulation occurs to cause contraction, the gallbladder tends to remain full and does not receive or concentrate new bile. In fact, the liver is not stimulated to produce bile if the gallbladder is full, resulting in nonvisualization of the gallbladder radiographically.

On the evening preceding the examination, the patient is given a fat-free supper, and the contrast tablets are taken. Tablets may be prescribed according to body weight and may vary in number from 6 to 12. They are taken one at a time, 5 minutes apart, with minimal water. After ingestion of the tablets the patient is NPO except for sips of water until the examination is completed.

A preliminary film is taken, processed, and evaluated before proceeding with the remainder of the study. This "scout" film has considerable technical value but is primarily used to determine whether or not the contrast medium is concentrated in the gallbladder. The study need not be continued if the gallbladder is not opacified.

In approximately 10% to 20% of oral cholecystograms, the gallbladder cannot be visualized on the first attempt. This may result from problems that could occur along the route of the contrast medium. For example, pyloric stenosis (stricture of the stomach outlet) may prevent the contrast medium from reaching the intestine. Occasionally a patient may experience nausea and vomiting after ingestion of the tablets. This may be a reaction to the contrast tablets but is often the typical response to a malfunctional biliary system.

In some patients, absorption in the small bowel may be limited because of coating of the intestines by mineral oil or laxative products containing oily substances. Absorption is also a problem in patients with "rapid transit syndrome," when food passes too quickly through the bowel because of irritation or other causes. If no problem exists in the gastrointestinal (GI) tract and absorption occurs as expected, the contrast medium may still be prevented from reaching the gallbladder because of liver problems. Liver disease, such as hepatitis or cirrhosis, may prevent extraction of contrast medium and inhibit bile production.

If a blood chemistry test has been done for bilirubin (bile content in the blood) before the gallbladder examination, one should check the results before proceeding with an oral cholecystogram. Normal bilirubin values range from 0.2 to 0.8 mg/dl. When the bilirubin value is greater than 1.5, the patient must receive medical management to bring the level to less than 1.5 before proceeding with the examination.

With good liver function the next stumbling block in the process of visualization could be the gallbladder itself. Severe inflammation may prevent the gallbladder from storing bile. An abundance of calculi may leave little or no room for bile in the gallbladder or may impair its function mechanically by blocking the opening to the cystic duct.

When little or no concentration of contrast medium is seen on the scout film, a second attempt at opacification may be made. It is common practice to refer the patient for ultrasound studies of the gallbladder. Often this procedure provides an immediate diagnosis, eliminating the need for further radiography. If a repeat x-ray study is desired, the patient must be maintained on a fat-free diet. An additional dose of contrast tablets is given in the evening, and another film is taken the following morning. If the liver or gallbladder is sluggish but functioning, the longer time and increased concentration of the contrast medium in the blood often allow at least faint visualization on the third day after the initial dose. Failure at this point is often attributed to a nonfunctional gallbladder if clinical signs do not indicate problems with either the liver or the GI tract.

When the gallbladder has been successfully demonstrated, a radiograph after a fatty meal may be indicated (Fig. 9-6). The patient is given an oral gallbladder stimulant, such as Neo-Cholex, and the gallbladder is radiographed again after 20 to 30 minutes. These films may be useful in demonstrating gallbladder function as well as in visualizing the cystic and common bile ducts.

Common bile duct examinations

At one time the intravenous cholangiogram (IVC) was the preferred method of examining the common bile duct, but a high degree of risk was associated with the IV contrast used. Today, percutaneous transhepatic cholangiography (PTC), T-tube cholangiography, and endoscopic retrograde cholangiopancreatography (ERCP) serve this purpose. Ultrasound examinations are also helpful in the diagnosis of some common bile duct problems.

Percutaneous transhepatic cholangiography. PTC, sometimes called *thin-needle cholangiography,* involves placing the tip of a long, thin needle directly into the common bile duct. From 20 to 40 ml of a multipurpose contrast medium of 50% to 60% strength is injected under fluoroscopic control for fluoroscopic and radiographic visualization of the biliary system.

The radiographer's role is to assist the radiologist with the skin preparation and sterile techniques required for penetration of the common bile duct and to complete the procedure's technical aspects.

PTC presents risk to the patient and is usually attempted only when immediate information is needed and more conservative approaches are not practical or have been unsuccessful. Possible complications include leakage of bile into the peritoneal cavity, hemorrhage, pneumothorax, and sepsis (infection).

T-tube cholangiography. After cholecystectomy, a tube is sometimes left in the patient temporarily. This flexible rubber tube is about the size of a drinking straw in the form of a T. The cross-bars of the T extend into the hepatic and common bile ducts. The base of the T extends through a small surgical hole in the common bile duct and out through a small opening left in the original incision.

The T tube serves primarily as a drain for bile until the postsurgical edema in the common bile duct subsides and bile can pass normally into the duodenum. It also serves a second purpose as an avenue for the administration of contrast medium if it is necessary to examine the biliary system postoperatively. This study may be performed to detect residual calculi in the hepatic or common

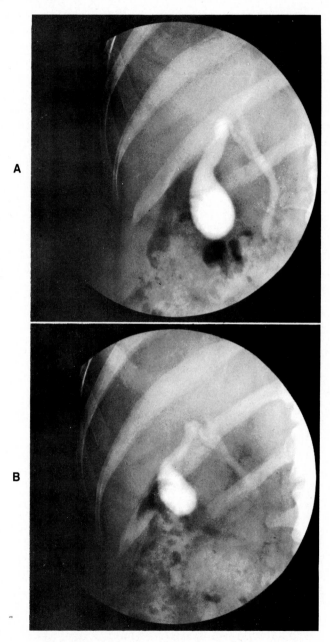

Fig. 9-6. Oral cholecystograms. **A,** Opacified gallbladder. **B,** After fatty meal. Note visualization of biliary ducts.

bile duct, but it is most frequently used to determine the patency of the ducts before removing the drain.

Often a T tube cholangiogram is performed in conjunction with the surgery to ensure that any remaining calculi in the ducts may be detected and removed before closing the incision (Fig. 9-7). In an operative study the T tube may or may not be left in place when the incision is closed.

During surgery the radiographer's duties are strictly technical. Patient care is accomplished by the anesthesiologist, and contrast injection is performed by the surgeon with assistance from the surgical nursing staff (see Chapter 10).

A postoperative study done in the radiology department requires that the radiographer assume a more prominent role. To accomplish this study, fill a 30 ml syringe with the contrast medium, a multipurpose aqueous iodine preparation such as Renografin-60 or Hypaque Meglumine 60%. Attach a 19-gauge butterfly set to the syringe, first filling the tubing with contrast medium and *eliminating all air from the tubing and the needle.* Air bubbles injected into the biliary system are often indistinguishable from residual calculi. Clamp the distal portion of the T tube off with a hemostat, and cleanse an area on the tube surface proximal to the clamp with an alcohol swab. Insert the needle into the T tube, and tape in place. The radiologist will inject the contrast medium under fluoroscopic control and take spot films of the biliary system.

You should review the contents and availability of the emergency supply kit before any procedure involving contrast, but reactions to this study are extremely rare compared with those involving IV injections.

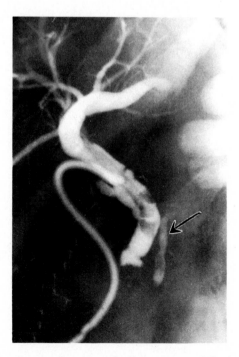

Fig. 9-7. T-tube cholangiogram showing calculi in common bile duct and visualization of pancreatic duct *(arrow).*

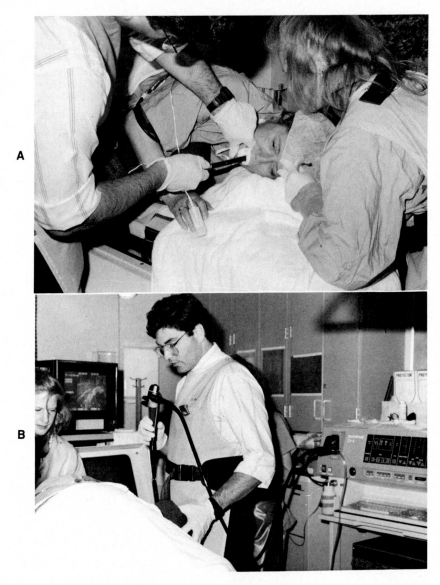

Fig. 9-8. **A,** Gastroscope placement for ERCP examination. **B,** Radiologist manipulates catheter through gastroscope under fluoroscopic control.

Endoscopic retrograde cholangiopancreatography.   ERCP is a fiberoptic examination of the common bile duct that uses an endoscope (gastroscope). The tu-
bular portion of the gastroscope is passed through the patient's mouth (Fig.
9-8) and through the stomach into the duodenum. A small catheter is then
passed through the gastroscope into the distal end of the common bile duct
through the papilla of Vater (Vater's ampulla). Contrast is injected through the
catheter under fluoroscopic control, with spot films to record the cholangiogram radiographically.

Attachments for the gastroscope include a "stone basket" for removal of biliary calculi and a tiny rotary blade for excising scar tissue or other obstructions.
Sometimes a small plastic tube called a *stent* is left in the papilla to facilitate bile
drainage.

This procedure may be performed in the radiology department or in a minor
surgical setting using the C-arm fluoroscope (see Chapter 10).

OTHER CONTRAST EXAMINATIONS

Myelography

The myelogram is an examination that uses contrast media to visualize the internal surfaces of the spinal canal. This study aids in the diagnosis of conditions
characterized by deformity or crowding of the spinal canal, such as spinal cord
tumors and intervertebral disc problems.

The injection procedure is called a *spinal tap* or *lumbar puncture* and involves
the insertion of a needle into the subarachnoid space. The contrast medium is
then injected through the needle.

The usual medium is an aqueous, non-ionic contrast agent such as Isovue-M.
The aqueous medium is miscible in spinal fluid and outlines the nerve roots as
the fluoroscopic table is tilted into various positions. Fluoroscopic spot films
record regions of interest. A CT study may follow the myelogram in order to
obtain axial images of the spinal canal while the contrast is present.

The aqueous contrast is readily absorbed from the spinal fluid and excreted
via the urinary tract. This characteristic is a disadvantage in a prolonged procedure because the contrast medium may begin to disappear before the study is
complete. For this reason, it is important to avoid delays between the time of
injection and the examination.

The radiographer's role during a lumbar puncture is to assist the physician.
In preparation, the radiographer needs to assemble the following items:
1. Sterile myelogram tray or lumbar puncture tray
2. Antiseptic for skin preparation (e.g., Betadine, Merthiolate)
3. Ample supply of the contrast medium
4. Sterile gloves to fit the physician (two pairs)
5. Sterile spinal manometer (if needed and not included on the tray)

When the necessary items are ready, the patient is positioned, according to
the physician's preference, either prone with a bolster under the abdomen or
laterally recumbent with the hips flexed and knees drawn up toward the chin.
In either position the objective is to provide convenient access to the puncture
site for the physician while providing maximum lumbar flexion to separate the
spinous processes at the level of the injection (Fig. 9-9). The site may be any

intervertebral interspace from the twelfth thoracic–first lumbar (T12-L1) through fifth lumbar–first sacral (L5-S1). The L2-L3 and L3-L4 interspaces are frequently used. The physician prepares the skin, drapes the area, and proceeds with the puncture.

If a sample of spinal fluid is removed, it is placed in specimen tubes. The radiographer is responsible for ensuring that the specimen and requisition form are delivered promptly to the laboratory. Often the radiographer delegates this duty to another member of the staff and continues to assist the radiologist. The person who delivers the specimen must be instructed *not* simply to place it in a receiving rack but to notify the medical technologist that a spinal fluid specimen has been delivered. This is very important because a delay in processing the specimen may invalidate the results.

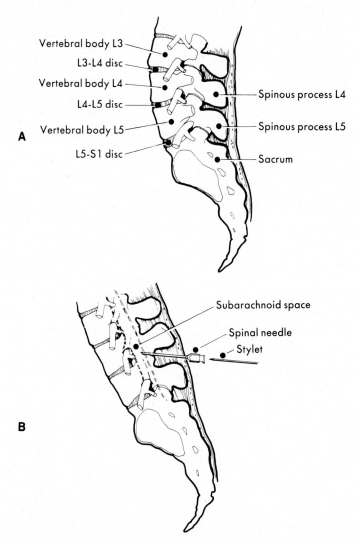

Fig. 9-9. Lateral aspect of lumbar spine. **A,** Normal posture. **B,** Spinal flexion separates spinous processes, allowing needle access to subarachnoid space.

The lumbar puncture procedure may also include the measurement of spinal pressure using a manometer. When this is done, the physician states the pressure readings aloud, and the radiographer records them for later inclusion in the chart and the radiologist's report.

When the physician is ready to make the injection, the radiographer opens the vial or ampule of contrast medium, shows the physician the label, and holds the container steady at a slight angle to facilitate withdrawal into the syringe.

After the injection the needle is withdrawn and the fluoroscopic examination proceeds.

The patient's head must be kept above the level of the spine, and the head of the radiographic table should not be lowered more than 15 degrees. You should check the footboard and shoulder guard on the fluoroscopic table to ensure they are secure before the table is tilted. During the examination, observe the patient for any change in appearance that might indicate a change in status. Listen for any complaint and provide reassurance. The patient may faint during the lumbar puncture or subsequent myelogram. Seizures and allergic reactions are rare but may occur at any time from the moment of injection to as long as 8 hours afterward.

Loss of spinal fluid with resulting lowered spinal fluid pressure tends to cause severe headaches following lumbar punctures. This discomfort is minimized by controlling activity and encouraging fluid intake for 24 hours after the examination. The patient is kept supine with head elevated 20 to 30 degrees for the first 8 hours, and activity may be restricted for a further 16 hours. Failure to keep the head elevated allows the contrast medium to flow upward to the hypothalamus, causing severe nausea with vomiting and potential dehydration.

Contrast arthrography

Arthrography, or contrast radiography of joints, is a special procedure used to detect injury and disease of the joint cartilage as well as abnormalities of the joint capsule (Fig. 9-10). The contrast medium for these studies may be a gas, one of the aqueous iodine compounds (50% to 60%), or a combination of both (double-contrast arthrography). The shoulder and knee are the most common sites of this study, but methods have also been developed for the study of the ankle and other joints arthrographically.

Patient care for these examinations consists mainly of providing explanation and support to the patient and assistance to the radiologist with the injection procedure. The necessary items are available commercially in a sterile disposable tray to which the radiographer must add disinfectant for skin preparation, contrast media, and gloves for the radiologist. The radiographer may also be called on to wrap the extremity with an elastic bandage after injection. This is done to maintain even pressure on the area for contrast localization and best visualization. The wrap must be firm but not tight. Periodically check the distal portion of the wrapped extremity for signs of decreased circulation. Coldness, numbness, discoloration, or swelling may indicate that the bandage is too tight. Bring any of these signs to the radiologist's attention. Fasten the bandage with adhesive tape rather than the usual metal clip, which is radiopaque and may obscure an anatomical area of interest.

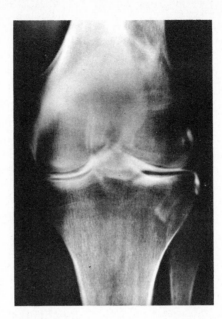

Fig. 9-10. Contrast arthrogram of knee.

Bronchography

Bronchography provides contrast visualization of the bronchial tree and is useful in the diagnosis and evaluation of such conditions as bronchiectasis, chronic pneumonia, hemoptysis, pulmonary tumors and cysts, and bronchial obstruction (Fig. 9-11). The use of bronchography has declined in recent years, since nuclear medicine and CT procedures provide improved diagnostic methods for many problems once investigated only with bronchography.

The contrast medium for this examination is a special preparation called Dionosil, which is available in both oily and aqueous solutions, the aqueous solution being more often used. Dionosil is very viscous at room temperature, so it is warmed to body temperature before the procedure by placing the vials in warm water. Dionosil also tends to separate on standing and must be thoroughly shaken before use.

Several methods may be used by physicians for the instillation of the contrast medium. In the *supraglottic method* the medium is rapidly dropped from a cannula onto the base of the tongue, with the patient's head in the vertical position. The contrast medium then flows posteriorly into the laryngeal orifice. The *intraglottic method* involves advancement of the cannula into the glottis. With the *intratracheal intubation method* a bronchial catheter is passed through the mouth or nose, through the glottis, through the trachea, and into the mainstem bronchus on the side of interest. In the *percutaneous cricothyroid* or *percutaneous transtracheal method* the trachea is entered directly with a puncture needle, either through the cricothyroid membrane or at an intercartilaginous space beneath it. This method is rarely used and requires that the patient be hospitalized.

In all the methods a local anesthetic is used to suppress the gag and cough reflexes, the contrast medium is instilled, and the patient's position is adjusted to promote gravity flow of the contrast agent into the various portions of the bronchial tree.

Careful preparation of the patient is essential to a successful bronchography examination. For the patient with an exudative lesion, the physician may prescribe an expectorant drug and postural drainage for several days before the examination. On the day of the examination the meal preceding the study is withheld, and the patient is NPO until 2 hours after the procedure. This precaution is taken to avoid the possibility of aspiration of food or fluid while the trachea is anesthetized. Sedation is given about an hour before the examination, and a drug such as epinephrine or atropine (to minimize bronchial secretions) is given approximately 30 minutes before examination.

The patient must be cautioned to suppress the cough reflex during the study, since coughing tends to remove contrast from the bronchi, forcing it back into the trachea as well as into the alveoli, where it diffuses and interferes with visualization of the bronchi. The patient should be reassured that he or she will at all times have adequate breathing space in the air passages and that the local anesthetic will help control the urge to cough. Patient cooperation is essential, and rapid, shallow breathing must be encouraged to keep the cough reflex under control.

Immediate follow-up care is provided in the radiology department. The pa-

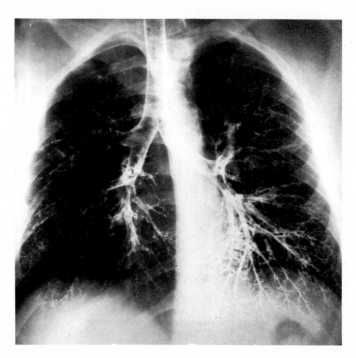

Fig. 9-11.   Bronchogram showing bronchial obstruction in left upper lobe. *(From Ballinger P: Merrill's atlas of radiographic and radiologic procedures, ed 7, St Louis, 1991, Mosby– Year Book.)*

tient is instructed to cough *gently*, which aids in the expectoration of the Dionosil, whereas forceful coughing tends to force it into the alveoli, where elimination by absorption takes a much longer time. Postural drainage aids in contrast elimination and is accomplished by reversing the positions used to fill the bronchi. A sitting posture is used to drain the upper bronchial segments, and the Trendelenburg position (supine with the head lower than the feet) is used to drain the lower segments. A postdrainage film is usually taken, following which inpatients may be returned to their rooms. Outpatients should be instructed to arrange to be escorted home to rest for the remainder of the day because of the prolonged effects of the sedation.

Angiography

Vascular radiographic procedures are collectively known as angiography and consist principally of arteriograms (studies of the arteries) and phlebograms or venograms (studies of the veins). Aqueous iodine compounds of various strengths are used for radiographic contrast, and a rapid series of films is taken using highly specialized equipment. The contrast medium used for angiography is chosen according to the requirements of the specific procedure (see Table 9-2). Many different technical procedures are included in this classification, since variations are necessary depending on the vessels to be visualized and the orientation of the radiologist or physician specialist who performs the injection. Vascular studies are one of the innovative frontiers of radiology, which explains why new methods are introduced at a rapid rate, and great diversity of method is found among departments. It is not necessary to explore all these variations individually, since most of them are quite similar from a patient care standpoint.

Percutaneous injection may be used for some angiographic studies, such as the extremities or the cerebral vasculature (Fig. 9-12). However, the preferred method of injection for most arteriography is with a catheter. Arteriographic catheters are radiopaque for visibility under the fluoroscope and come in a variety of lengths, gauges, and tip configurations to meet the requirements of various procedures.

Catheter insertion is accomplished by means of the *Seldinger technique*. A large artery, usually the femoral or axillary, is entered percutaneously with a large-bore needle. The needle is fitted with a stylet of equal length, which prevents blood from escaping back through the needle. When the needle is situated in the artery, the stylet is removed and a guide wire threaded through the needle and into the artery under fluoroscopic control. The needle is then removed, with the guide wire left in the vessel, and a catheter is threaded over the wire. The wire is then removed, with the catheter left in position for injection or further manipulation to engage selectively the vessel of interest.

For selective catheterization of smaller vessels, the catheter tip is maneuvered into the root of the vessel of interest, such as the coronary artery, a celiac artery, or a carotid artery (Fig. 9-13). A timed sequence of films is exposed after injection of the contrast medium, usually with the aid of an automatic power injector, which coordinates with the film changer and exposure control.

Computerized imaging equipment is used in many imaging centers to per-

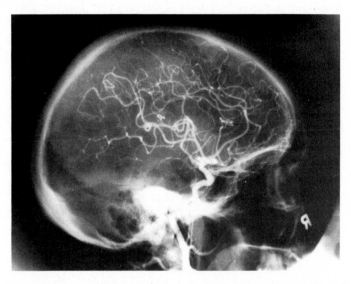

Fig. 9-12. Percutaneous cerebral angiogram. *(From Ballinger P: Merrill's atlas of radiographic and radiologic procedures, ed 7, St Louis, 1991, Mosby—Year Book.)*

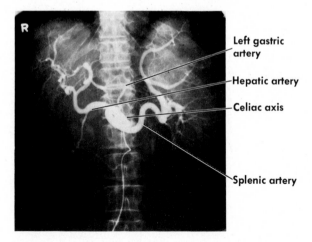

Fig. 9-13. Selective celiac arteriogram. Note catheter in abdominal aorta. *(From Ballinger P: Merrill's atlas of radiographic and radiologic procedures, ed 7, St Louis, 1991, Mosby— Year Book.)*

form digital subtraction angiography (DSA). Angiographic images are recorded by the computer on discs rather than on film. The images can then be manipulated, using the computer to enhance contrast and decrease the visibility of superimposing structures. The resulting computer images are recorded on film using a special camera. In some departments, DSA has completely replaced conventional film-screen angiography, especially for the cerebral vasculature.

DSA can be performed using either standard arteriographic catheterization or IV contrast injection. IV contrast administration obviously is less invasive than arterial catheterization and is therefore less hazardous. It is relatively painless and can be safely used in patients at high risk for arterial catheterization. IV contrast is less often used, however, because of the relatively poor anatomical detail obtained compared with arterial injections.

Patients are given preoperative medications before angiography and usually are sedated. Therefore, apprehension and anxiety are seldom problems at the time of examination. The patient usually is alert enough to cooperate in positioning but must not be left alone on the table.

The radiographer's role in any injection procedure is to be familiar with the radiologist's needs for equipment and supplies, to perform the skin preparation, and to assist with sterile technique. Specific training is needed to perform these functions because of the highly specialized nature of the procedures and equipment, but the basic principles of patient care and aseptic technique are the same as for other sterile injections and must be followed meticulously (Fig. 9-14).

After any arterial puncture, firm, continuous pressure is applied to the injection site for 5 to 10 minutes, followed by the application of a pressure dressing, which is monitored by the nursing service to avoid the possibility of hematoma

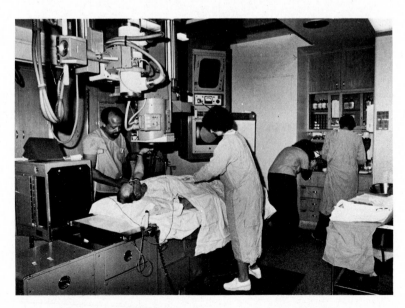

Fig. 9-14. Technologists prepare patient for angiography.

or hemorrhage. After studies that involve puncture of a vein, a pressure dressing is applied, and the patient may be discharged to resume normal activities.

SKIN PREPARATION

Procedures that involve puncture or incision of the skin require special skin preparation. Lumbar puncture for myelography and arterial catheterization for arteriography are typical examples of such procedures performed in imaging departments. The purpose of the skin preparation is to minimize the introduction of pathogens to the body via the puncture or incision, thus reducing the likelihood of infection.

Although it is not possible to sterilize the skin, a high degree of microbial dilution is accomplished by means of proper skin preparation. Preparation includes thorough cleansing, with hair removal if necessary, followed by application of an antiseptic solution such as Betadine or Zephiran and the surrounding of the prepared area with sterile drapes. The prepared area is usually a circle approximately 12 inches in diameter with the puncture or incision site at its center. The physician will specify the exact site.

Hair removal is not always required for skin preparation, and shaving is done *only* on the specific order of the physician in charge.

⟱ Preparing the skin for sterile procedures

1. Obtain a "skin prep set" and a bottle of antiseptic for painting the skin. The preparation set includes a basin, liquid soap such as pHisoderm, gauze sponges, razor, towel, forceps, and medicine cup.
2. Wash the hands.
3. Place the patient in a comfortable position and ensure privacy.
4. Explain what is to be done.
5. Expose an area slightly larger than the preparation site, keeping the patient as completely covered as possible to provide for comfort and modesty.
6. Fill the basin with warm water.
7. Using a gauze sponge, thoroughly wet the area to be shaved and apply soap, forming a lather. NOTE: If hair removal is not ordered, omit steps 7 to 10.
8. Shave a small area at a time. Hold the skin taut with one hand, and shave with short, firm strokes in the direction of hair growth. Rinse the razor frequently.
9. Rinse the area, removing all the hair.
10. Rinse and refill the basin with warm water.
11. Using soap and a fresh gauze sponge, cleanse the area completely. Starting at the puncture site, use a circular motion and scrub in ever-widening circles. Do not scrub harshly, but remember that friction is more effective than soap in cleansing the skin.
12. Use a sterile gauze sponge to remove the soap and water, again using a circular pattern and starting at the center. This pattern avoids recontamination of the area that has been cleansed.
13. Pour a little of the antiseptic into a waste container to cleanse the lip of the bottle.
14. Fill the medicine cup with antiseptic.

15. Grasp several gauze sponges with the forceps, and dip them into the antiseptic.
16. Paint the skin with the antiseptic, starting in the center of the area and working outward in a circular pattern. Discard the sponge.
17. Allow the skin to dry.
18. Repeat steps 16 and 17.
19. Open the pack containing the sterile drape or sterile towels. The physician, wearing sterile gloves, will drape the area surrounding the prepared site.

SPECIAL IMAGING TECHNIQUES

Up to this point we have mostly discussed examinations that every radiographer learns to perform, and the patient care procedures involved have been described in relative detail. The imaging techniques that follow are not found in every imaging department and are performed by radiographers with advanced training. These topics are introduced so that the beginning radiographer will have a general understanding of the nature and purpose of each and so that the safety procedures and patient care applicable to them can be highlighted. As a student you will want to know about these procedures so that you can provide preliminary explanations to patients who may come to your department to schedule appointments. You will also want to be prepared to assist with routine patient care if you have scheduled rotations into these specialty areas.

Computed tomography

CT is the same modality sometimes called computer-assisted tomography (CAT) scanning. The computer controls contrast levels, permitting a much greater degree of tissue differentiation than is possible with routine radiography. Axial images are made in slicelike sections in the transverse plane and may be "reconstructed" by the computer to display images in other planes as well.

The equipment (Fig. 9-15) consists of a movable table with remote control, a circular gantry structure that supports the x-ray tube and detectors, an operator console, supporting computer, magnetic tape drive for archiving data, and a computer-driven camera for committing the images to film. Additional consoles may provide remote viewing.

The diversity of CT is illustrated by the wide range of its applications, including studies of the brain, spine, abdomen, pelvis, chest, neck and paranasal sinuses. Orthopedic studies of the extremities may also use this method, and CT is useful in localizing both lesions and needle position during needle aspiration biopsies. It is a valuable tool for emergency use in the detection of intracerebral or intraabdominal hemorrhage.

Most CT examinations are noninvasive and are not uncomfortable for the patient. The equipment may cause apprehension, however, and careful explanations are necessary to obtain the patient cooperation that is essential to a satisfactory study.

Studies of the abdomen (Fig. 9-16) usually employ oral contrast to differentiate the GI tract from the surrounding tissues. A special barium compound (e.g.,

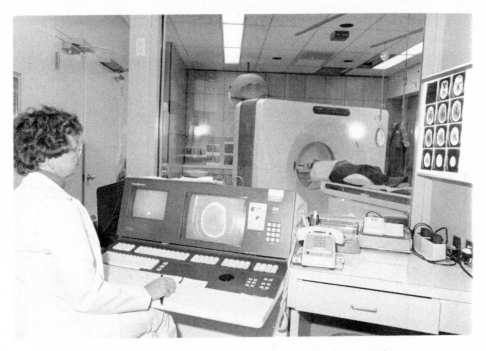

Fig. 9-15. Technologist observes patient from console during CT brain scan.

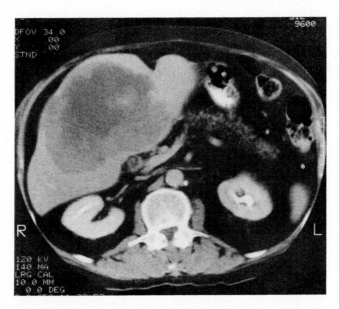

Fig. 9-16. Contrast-enhanced axial CT image of abdomen shows large liver lesion *(upper left)* and opacification of kidneys *(lateral to spine)*.

Baro-Cat) or an oral aqueous iodine medium (e.g., MD-Gastroview mixed with water and flavoring) is ingested by the patient over a period before the study. The amount of contrast and the time vary depending on whether the examination is to include the upper abdomen only or the entire abdomen and pelvis. For these studies the patient is instructed to fast before the procedure and to come early to drink the contrast preparation. Some departments may send the contrast home with the patient with instructions to drink it before reporting for the appointment.

IV injection of aqueous iodine contrast media (e.g., Conray-43, Isovue-200) may be employed to increase the contrast level of the patient's tissues. This is especially desired for studies of the chest, abdomen, and soft tissues of the neck, since it highlights blood vessels and vascular organs such as the liver and spleen. The contrast defines the renal collecting system, ureters, and bladder as it is excreted in the urine. Contrast is also employed to demonstrate brain lesions (Fig. 9-17).

Contrast administration may consist of a bolus of the medium injected rapidly at the start of the procedure and a continuation of the injection at a much slower rate as the examination proceeds. This can be accomplished by injecting the bolus with a syringe, followed by a drip infusion. Both can be accomplished by connecting the IV set to an automatic injector (Fig. 9-18) that can be programmed to provide the desired flow rates. This is the method most often used.

The IV line is established with a butterfly needle or intravenous catheter and then connected to the syringe, IV tubing, or injector tubing. A multiple injection port (heparin lock) or an established IV line with an injection port may be used for the injection. In this case, a needle (usually 18 gauge) is attached to the tubing or syringe and is used to penetrate the injection port. The injection port must first be cleansed with alcohol. Once situated, the needle is secured to the

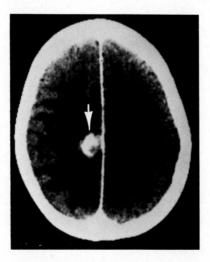

Fig. 9-17. CT brain scan with contrast enhancement. Arrow indicates metastatic brain tumor. *(From Ballinger P: Merrill's atlas of radiographic and radiologic procedures, ed 7, St Louis, 1991, Mosby–Year Book.)*

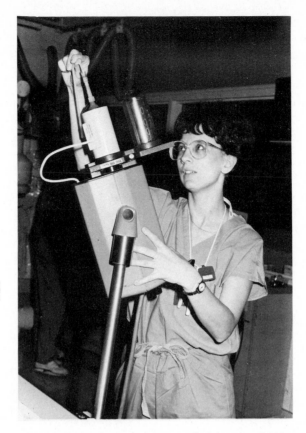

Fig. 9-18. Automatic injector controls contrast administration for CT examinations.

port with tape. If other IV fluids are being administered through the IV line, the tubing must be clamped off to stop the flow during the injection and released to restore the flow following the contrast injection.

The high volume of contrast used (often 200 ml) and the remote location of the technologist during the scan can create significant problems in the event of extravasation of the contrast medium. The use of a powerful automatic injector compounds this hazard. The following precautions will help minimize this risk:

1. Select an IV site other than an antecubital vein to avoid the possibility that elbow flexion will compromise the IV line. If an antecubital vein must be used, be careful that the arm is not excessively flexed. An arm board is recommended.
2. When using a heparin lock, flush before connecting it to the injection tubing to be sure the IV catheter is properly situated.
3. Double-check the IV site for possible extravasation at the time the automatic injector is started.
4. Instruct the patient to immediately report any sensation of burning, pressure, or other discomfort in the area of the IV site.

Review Chapter 6 for additional procedures and precautions related to IV injections.

MAGNETIC RESONANCE IMAGING

Magnetic resonance imaging (MRI) is a relatively new noninvasive diagnostic modality that does not use ionizing radiation. A magnetic field and pulses of radio waves are combined to produce a radio signal in the body that can be detected and computer processed to provide images on the computer monitor. The computer image may be stored on magnetic tape and is filmed with a special camera so that film copies are available for further study.

The MRI equipment includes a patient table, gantry (Fig. 9-19), and console combination with computer support. The gantry houses the magnet and is 5 to 6 feet long, surrounding most of the patient's body during the scanning process.

MRI provides excellent imaging of the soft tissues of the nervous system (Fig. 9-20) and is useful in the diagnosis of many types of pathology, including tumors of the brain and spinal cord, as well as diseases such as multiple sclerosis. MRI is being used increasingly in place of myelography for diagnosis of herniated intervertebral discs. This technique is also effective in imaging the soft tissue components of joints and is a reasonable alternative to arthrography of the knee, shoulder, and temporomandibular joint. One of the most recent advances in MRI technology is *magnetic resonance angiography* (MRA), which involves the study of the cardiovascular system.

Typical scan time for a series of slicelike images ranges from 2 to 20 minutes, and several series in different planes may be included in a typical examination. It is critically important that the patient remain still during a scan series and that the initial position be maintained throughout the study. Small movements, such as a cough or the chance to scratch the nose, may be permitted between series if necessary. Recent advances allow single images to be made in the space

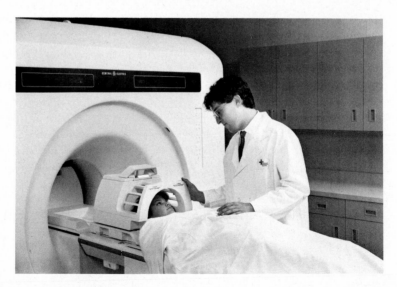

Fig. 9-19.   Patient receives reassurance before MRI examination of the brain. *(Courtesy Barrett Rudich.)*

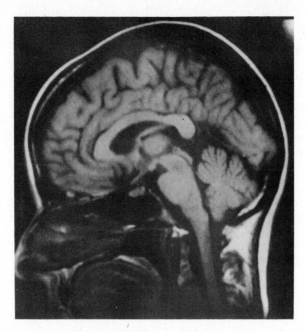

Fig. 9-20. Center sagittal MRI image of brain.

of a breathhold, allowing clear visualization of areas (e.g., liver) that would otherwise be blurred because of respiratory motion.

Although contrast agents are not required for most MRI studies, agents such as Magnevist (gadopentetate dimeglumine) and ProHance (gadoteridol), made from the rare-earth element gadolinium, are sometimes injected intravenously. These agents provide contrast enhancement of certain lesions, particularly brain and spinal cord tumors, and aid in differentiating disc material from scar tissue in postoperative studies of the spine.

Besides the IV injection of contrast agents, two patient care concerns are critical in MRI departments: (1) the effects of the magnet on objects within the room and possibly inside the patient's body and (2) helping the patient deal with anxiety about being placed in the close confines of the gantry, which may produce feelings of claustrophobia.

In addition to the magnetic field within the gantry, a fringe field exists within the room that may affect anyone who enters. Persons entering the room should first be interviewed to determine if they may have any surgical implants or metallic foreign bodies. Potential hazards exist from artificial heart valves, aneurysm clips, neurostimulators, middle ear prostheses, and intrauterine devices (IUDs). Cardiac pacemakers are a particular hazard, and *patients with pacemakers must not be permitted to enter the scan room.* Fatal incidents have occurred as a result of attempting to scan patients with pacemakers. Also of concern are patients who are pregnant or have hemolytic anemia, orthopedic pins and screws, or metal fragments or shrapnel in the soft tissues. Metalworkers who might have steel slivers in their tissues must have a screening radiographic or CT examination of the head to detect potential fragments that could damage their eyes or brain, since the pull of the magnetic field is so strong that it may influence the fragments to move. Patients are asked to remove makeup because metallic components may compromise the quality of the scan.

Caution is also needed to ensure that loose metal objects are not carried into the room. A pair of scissors, for instance, may fly from a pocket when entering the magnetic field, endangering bystanders and causing damage to the gantry. Even paper clips and hairpins can be hazardous. We especially want to caution you about entering the scanning room with stretchers, wheelchairs, or crutches that are not made especially for use with MRI, since *the magnetic field is sufficiently strong to pull these items out of control,* causing a serious accident. Steel oxygen tanks pose a great hazard and *must not* be taken into the scan room. Persons entering the scanning area should be cautioned not to bring watches, credit cards, hearing aids, or neurostimulators because the magnet will damage them.

Few people are completely comfortable for any length of time in a tightly enclosed space. Even patients with no history of claustrophobia may feel anxious on entering the gantry. Occasionally this anxiety is so severe that it amounts to panic, preventing the patient from continuing with the examination.

The radiographer can take several important steps to help the patient prepare for the examination and accept the emotional discomfort. An unhurried opportunity for the patient to survey the room can be coupled with an explanation of what to expect. The patient needs to know that he or she will lie on the table and that the table will move into the gantry. It helps to emphasize that plenty of air is available and that no physical discomfort will occur other than the need to lie still. The radiographer should also explain that the machine will make a loud "knocking" noise during the scanning process. Earplugs or earphones may be offered. Patients may be reassured to know that you will be communicating with them via an intercom and that you can hear them and see them at all times during the procedure. Since no danger exists from radiation, a friend or family member may be allowed to accompany the patient into the room and stay throughout the procedure if desired. Remember that *everyone* who enters the scan room must be screened for pacemakers, pregnancy, loose metal objects, and items that could be damaged by the magnet.

Often, claustrophobic patients do not have a rational explanation of their fears. It will help for them to focus their thoughts positively. Try asking what they like to do in their spare time. Suggest that they close their eyes and imagine that they are enjoying their favorite leisure activity during the procedure. Encourage them to enter the gantry, even for a few seconds, assuring them that they can come right back out if they wish to do so. After one successful trip in and out, most patients can control their anxiety sufficiently for the period required for one scan. It will help those who are still anxious to be brought out of the gantry between series so that the time spent in the confined space is minimized. When you are both patient and honest with claustrophobic patients, their confidence in you and in themselves will increase as the examination progresses successfully.

Claustrophobia sometimes necessitates the administration of a sedative in order for the patient to tolerate the procedure. Medications may also be needed for patients whose pain makes it impossible for them to lie still for the duration of the study. For these patients an IV catheter with intermittent injection port is established first. This provides access throughout the procedure in case it is needed for repeat doses, contrast administration, or emergency drug administration. The radiologist selects and administers the drug(s), and the technologist assists. Tranquilizers such as diazepam are frequently used to treat claustrophobia, and narcotics such as morphine or meperidine may be used for analgesia. Remember that these drugs act as respiratory depressants. The patient must be monitored with a pulse oximeter during the procedure because it is not possible to monitor the patient directly. Be certain that antagonists to reverse the effects of these drugs are available, as well as emergency supplies in the event of allergic reaction. (Review Chapter 6 for information on medication administration and sedation and Chapter 7 for responses to emergency situations.)

Diagnostic medical sonography

This imaging modality, often referred to as diagnostic ultrasound, uses high-frequency sound waves to produce echoes within the body. The strength and timing of the echoes' return to the sending point, or transducer, are interpreted by a computer to produce a map or graphic image of the echo distribution.

Any interface between substances or tissues of varying density produces an ultrasound echo. Sonography is a noninvasive technique that may be used to outline the shape and size of organs such as the spleen, gallbladder, or pancreas. Since it can distinguish fluid from adipose tissue, the presence of an abscess, tumor, or abnormal fluid such as ascites can be demonstrated.

Doppler methodology allows ultrasound recording of flow phenomena and permits demonstration of both arteries and veins. Vascular ultrasound is used extensively to detect arterial disease, particularly in the carotid arteries, and venous thrombosis of the extremities.

One of the more familiar uses of diagnostic sonography is the determination of gestational size for age of the fetus (Fig. 9-21). For this study the mother is requested to force fluids and not to void for 1 to 2 hours preceding the examination. This preparation provides a full bladder, which is the best "sonic window" for fetal imaging.

Nuclear medicine

A radioisotope or radionuclide is an unstable isotope that gives off radiant energy as its atoms decompose. Since isotopes enter into the same chemical reactions as their stable counterparts and are metabolized by the body in the same way, they can serve as tracers, which can then be followed and recorded by a gamma camera (Fig. 9-22). Abnormal tissues are demonstrated on the image because the isotope is metabolized at a different rate, at a different location, or to a greater or lesser extent than in normal tissue.

Where no suitable isotope exists to demonstrate a particular organ, a substance common to that organ can be "tagged" or "labeled" through a chemical process that binds it to a radioisotope. Technetium-99m (^{99m}Tc) is an isotope often used, both alone and in combination with other substances, because of its short half-life (6 hours) and because it is so versatile.

Structures that can be demonstrated by nuclear medical techniques include the thyroid gland, liver, lungs, brain, skeletal system, and kidneys (Fig. 9-23).

Special injection and disposal procedures required for the use of radioisotopes are beyond the scope of this text. For further information on this subject, consult a suitable nuclear imaging text.

Mammography

Mammography is a fairly routine radiographic procedure that uses special equipment and film to produce images of high contrast and high resolution for

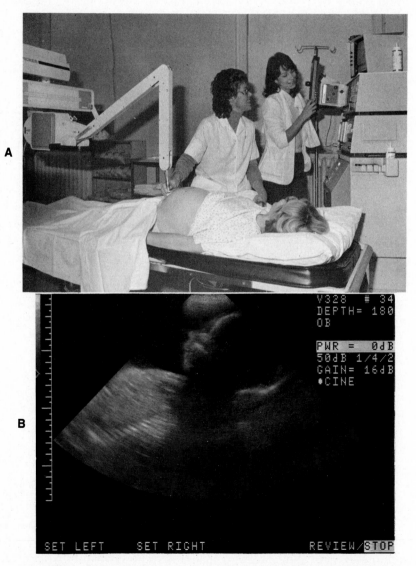

Fig. 9-21. Obstetrical sonography. **A,** Scanning procedure. **B,** Fetal sonogram.

diagnosis of breast lesions with little radiation dose to the patient. The American Cancer Society now recommends a baseline mammogram for women between the ages of 35 and 40, examination every 1 to 2 years between ages 40 and 50, and annual studies after age 50. Recent research in the field suggests that biennial mammograms after age 30 may soon be recommended for all patients, especially those with a family history of breast cancer.

Patients are instructed not to use underarm deodorant and not to apply powder or lotions on the breasts or axillary areas. These products may contain ingredients that produce artifacts on mammographic images. This is especially

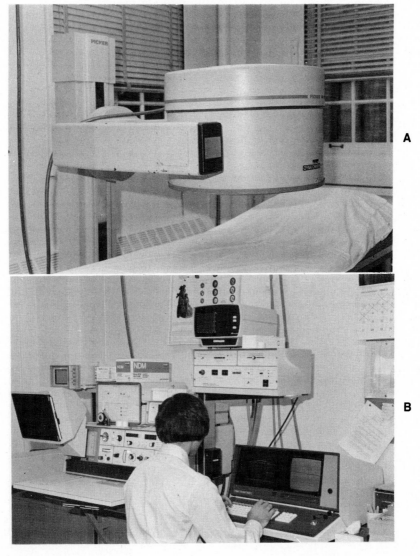

Fig. 9-22. Nuclear medicine laboratory. **A,** Gamma camera. **B,** Operator's console.

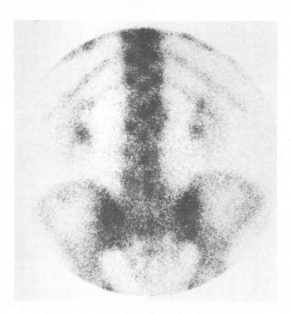

Fig. 9-23. Nuclear medicine scan of the lumbar spine.

true of antiperspirants that contain aluminum salts.

The mammographer obtains a pertinent history from the patient before the study. This usually includes the date of the last menstrual period, number of pregnancies, date of last pregnancy, whether the patient takes any hormones (including birth control tablets), and whether the patient has noticed any breast pain, breast lump(s), or nipple discharge. The precise locations of tenderness or lumps may be indicated on a breast diagram. When previous mammograms are available, every effort must be made to obtain them because comparative evaluation is often significant in the radiologic diagnosis.

Some departments include manual breast examinations during the mammography appointment. Mammography also provides an opportunity for patient instruction in breast self-examination (BSE).

Since the breasts must be uncovered for this examination, a comfortable temperature must be maintained in the radiographic room. To protect the patient's modesty, drape the upper torso with a sheet except during actual positioning and radiographic exposure (Fig. 9-24). Care must also be taken to avoid accidental intrusion by others during the examination. A simple door sign reading, "Examination in Progress: Do Not Enter," is very helpful.

Mammography units include a compression device that presses the breast tight against the film holder briefly during each exposure. Firm compression greatly improves the quality of the image for accurate interpretation and also reduces the amount of radiation necessary for an adequate exposure. Breast compression may be uncomfortable and may cause patients to be somewhat apprehensive but does not usually cause pain. Patients with very tender breasts, often from fibrocystic breast disease, may experience pain during compression

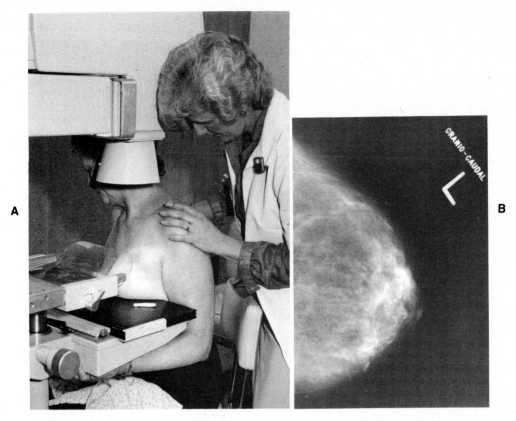

Fig. 9-24. Mammography. **A,** Positioning patient with mammographic unit. **B,** Low-dose film-screen mammogram.

or during the 24 hours that follow. Aspirin or acetaminophen is recommended for the treatment of postmammography pain.

In addition to routine screening examinations and studies for the evaluation of known breast lumps, mammographic techniques may also be used to localize needle placement for breast biopsies.

CONCLUSION

Radiographic examinations employing contrast media and special imaging procedures are used extensively in the hospital to enhance visualization of many soft tissue structures. Many media and methods are used, depending on the area to be radiographed and the individual policies of the department and the radiologist.

Contrast radiography provides opportunities for the radiographer to use skills developed throughout the study of patient care. These include providing explanations and reassurance, promoting asepsis, and communicating effectively.

Since there is potential danger of serious adverse reactions to contrast media, especially when injected intravenously, the radiographer must be prepared with equipment, supplies, and knowledge to deal with such occurrences and must be constantly alert to recognize early signs of allergic response.

Study questions

1. During an intravenous urogram, the patient becomes agitated and short of breath. What should you do?
2. Why is sterile technique important in cystography and catheterization techniques?
3. The preliminary film for an oral cholecystogram does not show opacification of the gallbladder. What should you do?
4. What considerations might cause anxiety in a patient undergoing a bronchogram? How can you help?
5. Why is it important for a radiographer to know about alternative imaging modalities, such as MRI and nuclear medicine?

Bedside Radiography: Special Conditions and Environments

Objectives

At the conclusion of this chapter, the student will be able to:

1. List three situations in which bedside radiography may be preferable to examination in the radiology department.
2. State the purpose of gastric, tracheal, and thoracic suction.
3. List precautions to be taken when doing a bedside examination of a newborn infant in the nursery.
4. List four important factors to be noted during an initial survey before radiography in the intensive care unit (ICU).
5. List three types of special beds or mattresses that may be seen in the ICU, and state the precautions to be used when doing mobile radiography with each type.
6. Discriminate between the terms *tracheotomy* and *tracheostomy,* and state three precautions to be taken with patients who have a tracheostomy.
7. Demonstrate the procedure for discontinuing gastric suction.
8. Define the term *sterile corridor,* and explain the significance of this concept to the radiographer.
9. State the consequences of dislodging a thoracic tube, and explain how to avoid this occurrence.
10. Demonstrate the appropriate procedure for gathering information before performing a bedside radiographic examination.

Vocabulary list

1. angiogram
2. atelectasis
3. dysplasia
4. enteric
5. hydrocephalus
6. ICU
7. Isolette
8. nasogastric
9. neonate
10. orthopedic
11. osseous
12. shunt
13. traction
14. ventilator

So far, we have discussed primarily patient care in the radiology department. This chapter deals with bedside radiography and fluoroscopy and with the conditions that are encountered when radiography is needed in other areas of the hospital. Emphasis is given to patient conditions that may be seen in critical care units but that may occasionally be encountered in the radiology department as well.

MOBILE RADIOGRAPHY

Hospital radiology departments are equipped with mobile x-ray generators. These are used primarily for bedside radiography and may also be used in the surgical suite. Studies done with this equipment are frequently called "portable" radiography examinations, but this is not a very accurate term. Portable means "capable of being carried," and few x-ray machines fit this description. When we mean to say "on wheels" or "capable of being moved around," mobile is the better word. Two types of units are generally used, the mobile radiographic unit and the C-arm mobile image intensifier, which is a fluoroscopic unit. The C-arm unit is also capable of producing radiographs of a relatively small anatomical area.

Bedside radiography is requested when a patient's condition makes it difficult or hazardous to transport the patient to the radiology department. Since mobile radiography equipment has significant technical limitations compared with the facilities in the radiology department, it is not always possible to do bedside examinations with the same ease and radiographic quality possible in the radiology suite. Therefore, the radiographer may consult with the nurse in charge regarding the advisability of doing a particular examination with mobile equipment. If it has been ordered as a mobile study by the attending physician, however, the examination must be done that way, or the physician's consent must be obtained to change the order if that course seems to be indicated.

Procedure

With the exception of chest radiographs, bedside examinations are seldom routine. Standard positioning may not be possible, and situations often demand creative, innovative approaches. The skills gained by observing and assisting experienced radiographers will help you learn to handle these difficult situations competently.

Except for "stat" or urgent requests, the radiographer should call the nursing service before leaving the radiology department to do a bedside examination. This will ensure that the patient is available for the examination and that radiography will not interrupt a meal, a bath, or a much-needed nap.

On arrival on the floor, check with the nurse in charge, make your presence known, and inquire about the patient's condition. With the permission of the nursing service, proceed to the patient's room. Do *not* push your equipment ahead of you as you enter. Park the machine outside, and enter alone first. Introduce yourself, explain the procedure to the patient, and move any obstacles out of the way before bringing the equipment to the bedside.

Bedside radiography may be requested for patients in isolation to avoid unnecessary contamination of the hospital or to protect the patient from possible infection from the hospital environment that could occur during transportation. If this is the case, you may wish to review isolation technique and procedures (see Chapter 5). The situations that follow represent other typical situations when bedside radiography may be advantageous.

ORTHOPEDIC TRACTION

Orthopedic traction is a mechanical method that uses weights to provide a constant pull, or traction, on part of the body for therapeutic reasons. In the past, fractured long bones such as the femur were placed in traction to maintain the alignment of bone fragments as they healed. More often today, traction is used only until muscle spasm subsides and the bone is surgically immobilized with a pin or plate. This permits a cast to be applied and releases the patient from the hospital to convalesce at home.

When you do encounter a patient in traction, remember that the sudden release of traction may result in serious harmful effects and should never be attempted by the radiographer. An accidental bump against the bed or the traction weights may cause severe pain. Since patients are usually aware of which motions are tolerable for them, one should allow the patient to assist as much as possible with any moving or lifting. Often the traction apparatus includes a trapeze bar that the patient may grip to assist in elevating the torso. If you have any doubt about the advisability of certain movements, obtain informed assistance from the nursing service.

SPECIAL CARE UNITS

The intensive care unit (ICU) is designed for patients in critical condition whose treatment and status require frequent monitoring. Depending on the size of your institution, intensive care could be subdivided into medical ICU, surgical ICU, coronary care, and so on. There may also be a trauma unit and neonatal and pediatric ICUs.

Intensive care units

The ICU is a familiar place to radiographers because many of these patients require monitoring radiographically. Since most ICU patients cannot be moved easily or safely to the radiology department, examinations are almost always done at the bedside. Chest films are most often called for, but other examinations may also be requested.

The inexperienced radiographer entering the ICU need not expect great difficulty in dealing with the acutely ill patient. Since there is always adequate staff to provide constant patient care, the radiographer's duties are limited almost exclusively to technical considerations. The special problems faced in this environment may be twofold: dealing with one's own anxiety at confronting near-death situations and dealing with an assortment of life-sustaining equipment connected to the patient or to other equipment by a network of cords, cables, pumps, and tubes (Fig. 10-1).

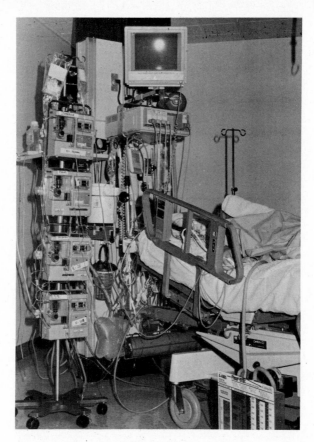

Fig. 10-1. Intensive care unit (ICU) may present bewildering array of pumps, monitors, cords, cables, and tubes. Can you identify the medication pumps? Closed chest drainage unit? Cardiac monitor?

Before bringing your equipment into the ICU, confer with the nurse in charge. The nursing service is familiar with the patient's condition and can provide both information and any assistance needed. Explain what you need to do to accomplish the procedure, and inquire about any special precautions that may be necessary. Next, assess the patient. Determine the degree to which the patient can cooperate with the procedure. If the patient is conscious, introduce yourself and explain what you plan to do. Even if the patient is not responsive, speak to the patient, providing a brief explanation and calm reassurance as you work.

Since space is sometimes limited, you may need to move some equipment to make room for the x-ray unit. Check the bed rails and the area under the bed to locate cords, tubes, and drainage receptacles so that you will be aware of their location and not damage them accidentally as you move equipment. Locate the most convenient electrical outlet, and decide just how and where you will place the x-ray unit. If the bed must be moved, obtain help from the nursing service. Usually two persons are needed to move the bed safely without placing undue stress on cables or tubes that are connected to the patient. Do not forget to place the lead shield in position for the protection of the staff and nearby patients.

When the plan is clear and the area is ready, bring in the x-ray unit and complete the study as efficiently as possible. When you have finished, be sure to return everything carefully to its original location.

Patients with ventilators, heart monitors, and other specialized equipment may be found in different parts of the hospital but are most frequently encountered in the ICU. Whatever their location, patients being monitored need the same precautions and attention to detail as those in a specialized unit.

Special beds and mattresses

Patients who are relatively immobile have problems with circulation in general, especially with skin integrity over any weight-bearing body surface. Many patients in both ICU and long-term care units share these problems. In the past it was customary to place immobile patients in beds or on frames that could be turned routinely to promote circulation and avoid the development of decubitus ulcers. New and innovative devices have made much of this equipment obsolete. Alternating pressure mattresses, rocking beds, and various types of wave, flotation, and bead mattresses are among the new types of equipment that enhance the well-being of patients who cannot tolerate being moved in the usual manner. The continual changes in position and pressure promote healing and avoid the need to turn patients from side to side.

When bedside radiography is needed for patients on special beds, consult the nursing staff to see exactly what equipment is being used. Beds that have a rocking motion or waves of alternating pressure need to be turned off during radiographic exposures to avoid motion blur on the radiograph.

Some patients are on a water-filled cooling mat to reduce body temperature. Since it is important to place the cassette on top of the mat to obtain the correct exposure, be careful not to snag the mat while positioning the cassette. The Mylar surface of warming blankets or pads is very effective in reflecting body heat back toward the patient's body. Again, you must place the cassette carefully between the patient's body and the reflecting surface without damaging the Mylar.

Tracheostomies

A tracheotomy is a surgical opening made into the trachea to create an artificial airway. When a tube is left in place to provide a temporary or permanent opening, it is called a tracheostomy (Fig. 10-2). A tracheotomy may be necessary due to obstruction in the upper respiratory tract, which may be caused by laryngospasm, cancer of the larynx, or burns in the mouth and throat. Another reason may be to provide controlled respiration with a ventilator in patients with respiratory collapse, such as paralysis, pulmonary edema, or chest trauma.

Most patients with a tracheostomy are in the ICU. If one of these patients must be brought to the radiology department, a nurse may be in attendance.

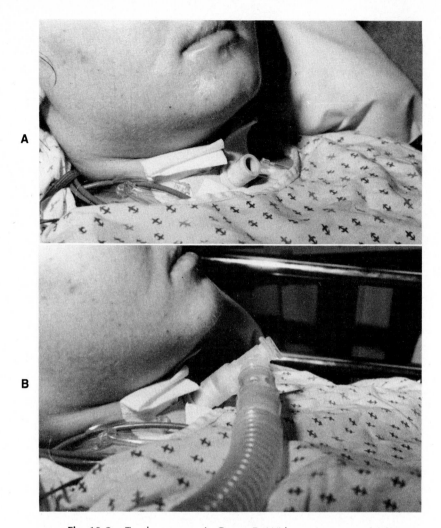

Fig. 10-2. Tracheostomy. **A,** Open. **B,** With respirator attached.

The most important factor to remember is never to untie the tapes holding the tracheostomy tube in place. A sudden cough can expel the tube, and the edges of the tracheotomy may close sufficiently to obstruct respiration. Patients who require frequent suctioning to keep the opening free of secretions must be kept under supervision where there is immediate access to suction equipment and sterile supplies.

Mechanical ventilation

Patients who need mechanical assistance with respiration are *intubated;* that is, a tube is passed through the mouth and into the trachea. The tube is then connected to a ventilator (mechanical respirator), which assists breathing, either by supplementing the patient's breath or by forcing respiration under pressure. Ventilators may also be connected directly to tracheostomies (Fig. 10-2, *B*).

When doing an examination of the torso, it is often desired to turn off the ventilator momentarily during the exposure to avoid motion blur on the radiograph. This should be done only with the knowledge and approval of the nurse in charge and only if you have been shown exactly how to do it. It is preferable to ask the nursing staff to assist with the handling of the ventilator during these procedures. If the ventilator is controlling both the rate and the volume of breathing, you may be able to determine, by paying attention to its rhythm, when a brief pause in respiration will occur. If the exposure time is short and your sense of rhythm is good, you will be able to take a motion-free exposure without turning off the ventilator.

Patients may also be ventilated manually using a bag that is squeezed regularly by hand to force respiration. This method is used briefly during the time between intubation and setting up the ventilator. Manual ventilation, often referred to as "bagging," is also used when the patient is transferred for diagnostic studies. Usually a nurse and a respiratory therapist or cardiopulmonary technologist are in attendance.

Nasogastric tubes

Another treatment situation that may be encountered in the ICU and elsewhere involves the nasogastric (NG) tube. This device may be placed to allow feeding of the patient directly into the stomach, for example, when a tracheostomy prevents normal swallowing. With patients who have had recent surgery or who have an ulcer or bowel obstruction, the NG tube, connected to a suction device, may be used as a means of emptying the stomach. Gastric suction does not need to be maintained continuously. It may be disconnected temporarily for a trip to the radiology department.

To discontinue gastric suction, first check with the nursing service. With their approval, if you are familiar with the procedure, turn off the suction. Clamp off the tube with a hemostat, and then disconnect the tube. Wipe the tube with a tissue or gauze sponge, then double the end and wrap the bent portion tightly with a rubber band so that it will not leak. Remove the hemostat, and tape or pin the loose end of the tube to the patient's gown to keep the tube from being pulled out of position by its own weight. Take care not to remove the gown without first remembering to unfasten the tube. It is very unpleasant for the patient to have the tube reinserted.

When doing bedside radiography of a patient with an NG tube, little cause exists for concern except to take care not to disturb the tube. It is uncomfortable when tugged on and very messy if the drainage end is dislodged from the bottle or the suction machine.

A Levin tube is a short NG tube that goes only as far as the stomach. Nasoenteric tubes (Fig. 10-3) go further into the intestinal tract to aspirate gas and fluid that may cause distention postoperatively. This is also a frequent method of treatment for bowel obstruction. Some typical nasoenteric tubes are Miller-Abbott, Harris, and Cantor tubes. They are frequently localized radiographically. If passing a long tube beyond the stomach is difficult, the patient may be brought to the radiology department for manipulation of the tube under fluoroscopic control.

NG tubes may be used to instill contrast media into the stomach for radio-

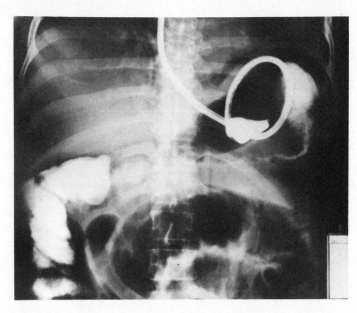

Fig. 10-3. Miller-Abbott tube used to treat small bowel obstruction. In this patient, tube is coiled within stomach.

graphic examinations. A thin barium mixture or oral aqueous iodine solution can be drawn up into a large syringe, which is then connected to the NG tube. The radiologist instills the contrast under fluoroscopic control. Oral contrast mixtures for CT examinations may also be instilled through the NG tube. This is done in advance of the examination by the nursing service.

Closed chest drainage

Closed chest drainage is a method used to remove fluid or air that has accumulated in the pleural space. It consists of a tube placed within the pleural cavity (Fig. 10-4) and connected to a suction device through a drainage receptacle. Note Pleur-Evac unit on floor near the foot of the bed in Fig. 10-1. Disturbance of this system at either end may result in a rush of air into the pleural space, reversing the intent of the treatment and possibly causing collapse of a lung. Extra caution is therefore required to see that the suction and drainage apparatus is not disturbed in the course of your work and that the chest tube is not dislodged in the process of positioning the cassette for a chest radiograph.

Specialty catheters

The radiographer encounters a variety of catheters with specialized functions that have been developed to aid in the monitoring and management of critical patients and those requiring long-term care. The precise nature and function of each of these catheters form a large, complex, rapidly changing body of information. Some of the names you may encounter are Swan-Ganz, Hickman,

Groshong, and Medi-Port. This is another area in medicine accurately described as an innovative frontier. In general, we refer here to tubes that provide access to the circulatory system on a repeated or continuing basis. There are many reasons why such access might be desired.

Pulmonary artery flow-directed catheters (e.g., Swan-Ganz) are used to diagnose right and left ventricular failure and pulmonary disorders and to monitor the effects of specific medications on heart function. These catheters are often seen in ICU patients who have undergone open heart or chest surgery and those who require intensive monitoring.

Chemotherapy or other long-term drug therapy may be facilitated by access to the central venous system for drug administration (e.g., Medi-Port). Kidney dialysis may use a catheter system until a shunt for permanent access can be established. Patients requiring long-term parenteral nutrition can now be treated at home through central venous catheters (e.g., Hickman). Some specialty catheters have multiple lumina that allow for many distinct functions. The access end of these catheters is usually located in the arm, neck, or shoulder. The distal end is located appropriately according to its purpose, perhaps in the pulmonary artery for pressure monitoring or in the supraclavicular vein for

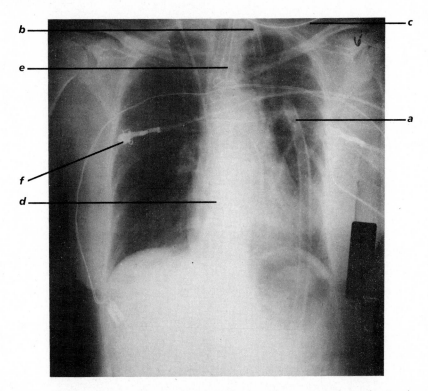

Fig. 10-4. Chest radiograph of patient with multiple catheters and electrodes in place. **A,** Pulmonary catheter for closed chest drainage. **B,** Tracheostomy tube. **C,** Oxygen catheter to tracheostomy (external). **D,** Central venous pressure monitor (CVP line). **E,** Nasogastric tube. **F,** Electrodes and leads for cardiac monitor (external).

medication administration (Fig. 10-5). Many of these systems use pumps and filters, which add to their usefulness.

The physical status of patients with specialized catheters may be placed in jeopardy by improper use of the catheter. For example, many medications compromise a parenteral nutrition line. Therefore, only personnel trained in their use are permitted access to these catheters.

Depending on type, specialty catheters may be inserted via venipuncture using a stainless-steel needle and guidewire or may be placed surgically via a cut-down procedure. Tip placement is often guided fluoroscopically in the cardiovascular laboratory or with the aid of a C-arm unit. New cardiac/intensive care units have beds designed to accept the use of C-arm fluoroscopes. This permits localization and possible realignment of catheters and tubes without transferring patients from their beds.

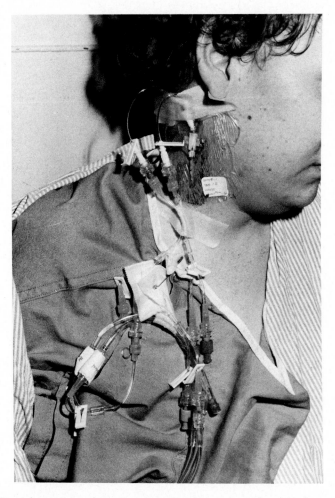

Fig. 10-5. Central venous catheter in supraclavicular vein with multiple access ports for medication administration.

Pacemakers

The pacemaker is an instrument that regulates the heartbeat by providing a minute electrical stimulation directly to the heart muscle, very similar to the stimulation normally provided by a nerve impulse. Internal pacemakers are surgically implanted within the patient's chest; external pacemakers are usually temporary measures, and the bulk of the instrument remains outside the patient's chest. When the pacemaker is inserted under fluoroscopic control, a radiographer is part of the team and may assist the cardiologist with some of the nursing procedures involved as well as with the technical aspects of fluoroscopic imaging. Depending on the facility, equipment available, and requirements of the individual patient, pacemakers may be inserted in the radiology department, operating room (OR), ICU, or coronary care unit. When fluoroscopy is required outside the radiology department, the equipment used is a C-arm fluoroscope.

Although the latest pacemaker catheters are nonconductive and therefore much safer for the patient, earlier catheters were capable of transmitting tiny electric currents. Improperly grounded equipment or even static charges from the bodies of health care workers could produce a *microshock*, which was carried by the catheter to the heart, causing fatal or very serious changes in heart function. Modern cardiologic technique has largely eliminated this hazard, but the radiographer should still be aware of the potential danger and ensure that all equipment used for such patients is in good repair and properly grounded.

NEONATAL NURSERY

Although most infants arrive in perfect health, newborns can have serious problems, and these patients are often monitored radiographically. For example, newborn atelectasis (failure of the lungs to expand completely) may require chest films for evaluation. Congenital hip dysplasia and possible fractures from birth trauma may indicate the need for osseous studies. Hydrocephalus (excess fluid in the ventricles of the brain) may require skull radiography to establish baseline information.

The premature infant is often placed in an Isolette (Fig. 10-6). This closed environment provides extra warmth, moisture, and oxygen while reducing the possibility of airborne infection as the infant gains maturity and strength. Some infants may be safely removed from the Isolette for brief periods and can be examined radiographically on an open table. The neonate at risk must be radiographed within the Isolette (Fig. 10-7).

Although there has been a recent trend toward less isolation for newborns, premature infants and those with health problems requiring radiographic examinations may still need protective precautions to avoid nosocomial infections. Protective precautions are described in Chapter 5. Even when sterile equipment and supplies are not required, attention to general principles of medical asepsis is essential to ensure the infant's safety.

A nursing staff member usually assists the radiographer. The cassette is covered and placed under the patient by the nurse, who positions the patient according to the radiographer's instructions. A short length of stockinette may be

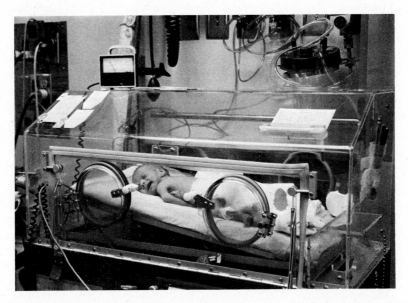

Fig. 10-6. Isolette provides warmth, moisture, and oxygen while premature infant gains maturity and strength.

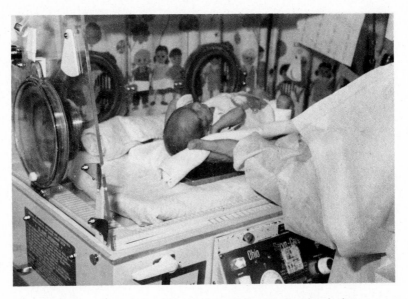

Fig. 10-7. Neonate at risk must be radiographed within Isolette.

slipped over the arms and/or legs to aid in immobilizing and positioning (see Chapter 3). For reasons of radiation safety, every effort should be made to stabilize the position so that the nurse need not hold the infant during the exposure.

SURGICAL SUITE

Surgical access and clothing

The radiographer also often works in the surgical suite. For reasons of asepsis, all traffic is controlled in the surgical suite. Access is limited to those persons and items that have a legitimate reason to be there. The inexperienced radiographer is not sent to the surgical suite alone for the first few visits. An experienced guide is essential to proper orientation.

Just inside the limited access area is a dressing room where one may change into surgical attire (Fig. 10-8), often called "scrub clothes." Beyond this point, access is allowed in scrub clothes only. On entering the surgical suite, you must wipe down the mobile x-ray machine with a germicidal solution before proceeding further. In some hospitals a mobile x-ray machine is maintained for surgical use only. Some surgical suites also have permanent radiographic installations. These measures help to reduce contamination in the OR. However, the radiographer must still be responsible for the equipment's cleanliness.

One must not go outside the surgical suite in scrub clothes. If you should have to leave, for example, to show a film to the radiologist, your clothes must be changed again before reentering the OR. This may be avoided by covering the scrub clothes with a long-sleeved gown when outside the surgical suite (Fig. 10-9).

Surgical setup

Some ORs have permanently installed x-ray equipment. When mobile equipment is used, it is usually kept outside the door until the moment films are desired (Fig. 10-10). For some procedures, however, the equipment may be positioned in advance and the tube head covered with sterile drapes during the setup. You must be familiar with the institution's policies and the surgeon's preferences.

When working in the OR, you must be aware of sterile fields and use caution not to contaminate them with your clothing or the equipment. The area between the patient drape and the instrument table is maintained as a "sterile corridor" (Fig. 10-11) and is the province of the surgeon and the instrument nurse only. Access to this area is permitted only to those persons wearing sterile gowns and gloves, and the radiographer is excluded from this part of the room. For abdominal surgery and open reduction of the lower extremities, the head end of the table is *not* a sterile field. This is a safe area from which the radiographer may assess the situation from a technical viewpoint. Cassettes are sometimes positioned via a tunnel in the operating table that may be reached from the nonsterile area. Otherwise, they are placed in a sterile cover and positioned by the surgeon. The technique of cassette transfer to a sterile cover is the same as that used for protective precautions (see Chapter 5).

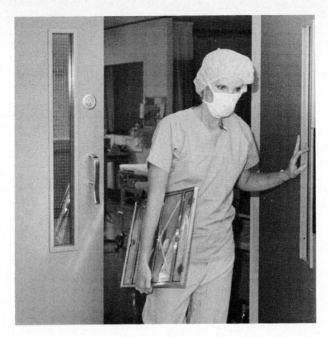

Fig. 10-8. Radiographer leaves surgical dressing room in "scrub clothes."

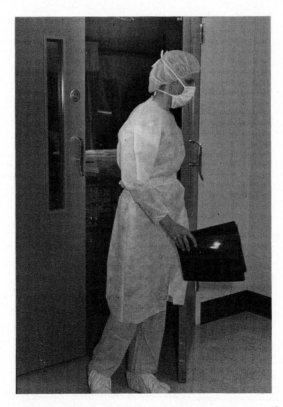

Fig. 10-9. Radiographer covers scrub clothes when leaving surgical suite temporarily. Gown is removed on return to surgery.

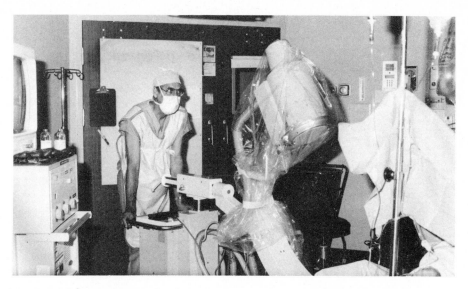

Fig. 10-10. Radiographer carefully moves C-arm mobile fluoroscope into position in operating room. Note wrapping of image intensifier to prevent possible contamination of sterile field by dust from equipment.

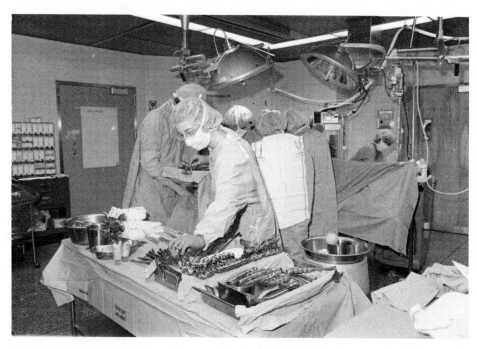

Fig. 10-11. Operating room during surgical procedure. Can you identify sterile corridor?

Surgical procedures often requiring radiography

One study performed by the radiographer in the surgical suite is the surgical cholangiogram, a frequent adjunct to cholecystectomy. The basis for this radiographic examination is explained in Chapter 9 as part of the discussion on T-tube cholangiography. When surgical cholangiograms are anticipated, the radiographer may be notified to come to surgery before the sterile field is established. At this stage the radiographer can locate anatomical landmarks and determine the correct film tunnel location for cassette placement. A preliminary film verifies that correct film location and technical exposure factors have been established before the patient is anesthetized and draped. Advance preparation permits the radiographer to proceed quickly and accurately later when the surgeon is waiting for results. This avoids delays that may increase patient risk by prolonging the anesthesia time.

If a preliminary film is not taken, the radiographer uses patient height and weight data to estimate exposure factors and relies on the surgical team to indicate the centering point for film and x-ray tube placement. In some institutions these methods are believed to be sufficiently reliable, and the preliminary film is not a part of the usual routine. The C-arm unit is sometimes used for surgical cholangiograms.

Another common surgical application of radiography is the open reduction of fractures. Plaster or fiberglass casts are used to hold many fractures in position while healing occurs. Some fractures, however, require surgical intervention to align the fragments. Internal fixation by means of rods, nails, plates, or screws is used to maintain the alignment securely. This method is often used to stabilize fractures of the hip and may be used for many other types of fractures as well. Reconstructive orthopedic surgery to correct crippling from developmental defects, previous injuries, or degenerative diseases may also require imaging. A radiographer may be present during these procedures, using the C-arm unit to provide fluoroscopic guidance for aligning bone fragments and placing hardware. A radiographic record is made of the final position of the bones and fixation devices.

Localization is the reason for several types of surgical radiography. Radiographs or fluoroscopic visualization may help in determining the exact location of foreign bodies such as bullets, sewing needles, or industrial steel fragments during their surgical removal. A spinal needle may be positioned in a spinal disc space and radiographed to establish the accuracy of the spinal level before proceeding with surgical intervention. A radiograph may be used to locate a surgical sponge or instrument within the abdominal cavity if the surgical count indicates a missing item before final closure of the incision. C-arm fluoroscopy may guide the surgical placement of internal pacemakers or catheters. Ultrasound is used in surgery for precise localization of tumors in the brain, spine, and liver.

Surgical environment

The surgical suite may seem to have a mysterious quality. One reason for this may be that there is usually a great deal of activity with very little noise. Sudden noises or loud conversations are distracting to the surgical team and may make it difficult for the anesthesiologist to hear heart sounds. Remember, the surgical patient is always at risk to some degree. This fact places pressure on the surgical team to work quickly.

A surgical team works best in a low-key environment and strives to maintain this type of atmosphere. The tension level may escalate, however, when things are not going well or when errors cause delays. You know how difficult it is to wait patiently when you are tense and anxious. This may be the state of mind of the surgeon and surgical staff as they wait for you to set up equipment, take radiographs, and process the films. Their work is "on hold," since they cannot proceed without the information your films will provide. When the stress level is high, they may urge you to hurry or may show an impatient attitude or tone of voice. At these times the ability to proceed confidently and speak calmly will help insulate you from the stress and will allow you to complete your work quickly and accurately.

CONCLUSION

Radiography at the bedside and in surgery takes the radiographer out of the radiology department and into the hospital's larger environment. Patients seen under these circumstances may be in critical condition or may be in the process of undergoing special treatments that require the radiographer's understanding and caution.

When working in other departments, the radiographer must respect the rules and wishes of the personnel in charge, communicate clearly, and obtain any information that may be lacking before proceeding. These situations provide some of the most interesting and challenging opportunities to the radiographer.

Study questions

1. How does mobile radiography differ from conventional radiography? Are any special skills required?
2. How would you prepare to take a chest radiograph on a patient in the ICU?
3. What precautions should be taken with a patient who has a tracheostomy?
4. What precautions are necessary when making a chest radiograph on a patient with closed chest drainage? Why?
5. How should a radiographer approach the patient for an abdominal film in surgery? What might be a good location for the control portion of the mobile x-ray machine?

References

APIC guidelines for infection control practice, Association for Practitioners in Infection Control, Inc, January 1990.

Ballinger PW: *Merrill's atlas of radiographic positions and radiologic procedures*, ed 7, St Louis, 1991, Mosby.

Blumenreich GA: The standard of care, AANAJ 59(4):302-304, 1991.

Brown M: How do you spell assessment? *Am J Nurs* 91(2):55-56, 1991.

Carnerie F: Violence against nurses: a pound of prevention is worth a pound of cure, *Registered Nurse* 2(1):42-43, 1990.

Colandrino C: Barium enema procedure for the pediatric patient, *Radiol Technol* 60(3), 1989.

Dowd SB: AIDs, the technologist and universal precautions, *Radiol Technol* 62(4), 1991.

Dowd SB: The radiographer's role: part scientist, part humanist, *Radiol Technol* 63(4), 1992.

Finesilver C: Respiratory assessment, *RN* 55(2):22-30, 1992.

Green E et al: Charting the future of emergency drug protocols, *Nurs '92* 22(6), 1992.

Hill MN, Grim CM: How to take a precise blood pressure, *Am J Nurs* 91(2):38-42, 1991.

Levesque TM: Applying therapeutic communications, *RT Image* 6(31):36-38, 1992.

Malasanos L et al: *Health assessment*, ed 3, St Louis, 1986, Mosby.

O'Brien L, Bartlett K: TB plus HIV spells trouble, *Am J Nurs* 92(5):28-34, 1992.

Plumer AL: *Principles and practice of intravenous therapy*, ed 4, Boston, 1987, Little, Brown.

Potter PA, Perry AG: *Basic nursing procedures*, ed 2, 1991, St Louis, Mosby.

Potter PA, Perry AG: *Fundamentals of nursing*, ed 2, 1990, St Louis, Mosby.

Silberman J: Patients have rights too, *US News World Rep* 5(2):59-64, 1990.

Sounesso G: Pulse oximetry, *Nurs '91* 21(8):60-64, 1991.

Tingle J: Nurses and the law: the right to confidentiality, *Nurs Times* 86(35):58-59, 1990.

Wavelength Reports: Health care workers protected from HIV/HBV by OSHA rule, *RS Wavelength* 3(8):10, 1992.

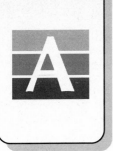

A Model Patient's Bill of Rights*

1. The patient has a legal right to informed participation in all decisions involving his health care program.
2. We recognize the right of all potential patients to know what research and experimental protocols are being used in our facility and what alternatives are available in the community.
3. The patient has a legal right to privacy respecting the source of payment for treatment and care. This right includes access to the highest degree of care without regard to the source of payment for that treatment and care.
4. We recognize the right of a potential patient to complete and accurate information concerning medical care and procedures.
5. The patient has a legal right to prompt attention, especially in any emergency situation.
6. The patient has a legal right to a clear, concise explanation of all proposed procedures in layman's terms, including the possibilities of any risk of mortality or serious side effects, problems related to recuperation, and probability of success, and will not be subjected to any procedure without his voluntary, competent, and understanding consent. The specifics of such consent shall be set out in a written consent form signed by the patient.
7. The patient has a legal right to a clear, complete, and accurate evaluation of his condition and prognosis without treatment before he is asked to consent to any test or procedure.
8. We recognize the right of the patient to know the identity and professional status of all those providing service. All personnel have been instructed to introduce themselves, state their status, and explain their role in the health care of the patient. Part of this right is the right of the patient to know the physician responsible for his care.
9. We recognize the right of any patient who does not speak English to have access to an interpreter.

---

*From Annas GJ: *The rights of hospital patients: an American Civil Liberties Union handbook,* New York, 1975, Avon.

10. The patient has a legal right to all the information contained in his medical record while in the health care facility and to examine the record upon request.
11. We recognize the right of a patient to discuss his condition with a consultant specialist at his own request and his own expense.
12. The patient has a legal right not to have any test or procedure, designed for education purposes rather than his direct personal benefit, performed on him.
13. The patient has a legal right to refuse any particular drug, test, procedure, or treatment.
14. The patient has a legal right to both personal and informational privacy with respect to the hospital staff, other physicians, residents, interns and medical students, researchers, nurses, other hospital personnel, and other patients.
15. We recognize the patient's right of access to people outside the health care facility by means of visitors and the telephone. Parents may stay with their children and relatives with terminally ill patients 24 hours a day.
16. The patient has a legal right to leave the health care facility regardless of physical condition or financial status, although he may be requested to sign a release stating that he is leaving against the medical judgment of his physician or the hospital.
17. No patient may be transferred to another facility unless he has received a complete explanation of the desirability and need for the transfer, the other facility has accepted the patient for transfer, and the patient has agreed to transfer. If the patient does not agree to transfer, the patient has the right to a consultant's opinion on the desirability of transfer.
18. A patient has a right to be notified of discharge at least 1 day before it is accomplished, to demand a consultation by an expert on the desirability of discharge, and to have a person of the patient's choice be notified.
19. The patient has a right, regardless of source of payment, to examine and receive an itemized and detailed explanation of his total bill for services rendered in the facility.
20. The patient has a right to competent counseling from the facility to help him obtain financial assistance from public or private sources to meet the expense of services received in the institution.
21. The patient has a right to timely prior notice of the termination of his eligibility for reimbursement for the expense of his care by any third-party payer.
22. At the termination of his stay at the health care facility, we recognize the right of a patient to a complete copy of the information contained in his medical record.
23. We recognize the right of all patients to have 24-hour-a-day access to a patient's rights advocate, who may act on behalf of the patient to assert or protect the rights set out in this document.

Informed Consent
Form

Southwest Washington Medical Center
VANCOUVER, WA

SPECIAL CONSENT TO OPERATION, POST OPERATIVE CARE, MEDICAL TREATMENT, ANESTHESIA, OR OTHER PROCEDURE

Patient: _____   Patient No. _____

Washington State law guarantees that you have both the right and obligation to make decisions concerning your health care. Your physician can provide you with the necessary information and advice, but as a member of the health care team, you must enter into the decision making process. This form has been designed to acknowledge your acceptance of treatment recommended by your physician.

1. I hereby authorize Dr. _____
   and/or such associates or assistants as may be selected by said physician to treat the following condition(s) which has (have) been explained to me: (Explain the nature of the condition(s) in professional and lay language.)

   _____
   _____
   _____

2. The procedures planned for treatment of my condition(s) have been explained to me by my physician. I understand them to be: (Describe procedures to be performed in professional and lay language.)

   _____
   _____
   _____
   _____

   At: _____
   (NAME OF HOSPITAL OR MEDICAL FACILITY)

3. I recognize that, during the course of the operation, post operative care, medical treatment, anesthesia or other procedure, unforeseen conditions may necessitate additional or different procedures than those above set forth. I therefore authorize my above named physician, and his or her assistants or designees, to perform such surgical or other procedures as are in the exercise of his, her or their professional judgment necessary and desirable. The authority granted under this paragraph shall extend to the treatment of all conditions that require treatment and are not known to my physician at the time the medical or surgical procedure is commenced.

4. I have been informed that there are significant risks such as severe loss of blood, infection and cardiac arrest that can lead to death or permanent or partial disability, which may be attendant to the performance of any procedure. I acknowledge that no warranty or guarantee has been made to me as to result or cure.

IMPORTANT: HAVE PATIENT SIGN FULL OR LIMITED DISCLOSURE BOX AND SIGNATURE LINE AT BOTTOM.

Full Disclosure

I certify that my physician has informed me of the nature and character of the proposed treatment, of the anticipated results of the proposed treatment, of the possible alternative forms of treatment; and the recognized serious possible risks, complications, and the anticipated benefits involved in the proposed treatment and in the alternative forms of treatment, including non-treatment.

_____
PATIENT/OTHER LEGALLY RESPONSIBLE PERSON SIGN
IF APPLICABLE

Limited Disclosure

I certify that my physician has explained to me that I have the right to have clearly described to me the nature and character of the proposed treatment; the anticipated results of the proposed treatment; the alternative forms of treatment; and the recognized serious possible risks, complications, and anticipated benefits involved in the proposed treatment, and in the alternative forms of treatment, including non-treatment.

I do not wish to have these risks and facts explained to me.

_____
PATIENT/OTHER LEGALLY RESPONSIBLE PERSON SIGN
IF APPLICABLE

Any sections below which do not apply to the proposed treatment may be crossed out. All sections crossed out must be initialed by both physician and patient.

5. I consent to the administration of anesthesia by my attending physician, by an anesthesiologist, or other qualified party under the direction of a physician as may be deemed necessary. I understand that all anesthetics involve risks of complications and serious possible damage to vital organs such as the brain, heart, lung, liver and kidney and that in some cases may result in paralysis, cardiac arrest and/or brain death from both known and unknown causes. I understand there is a risk of dental injury during airway management.

6. I consent to the use of transfusion of blood and blood products as deemed necessary, and potential complications associated with this procedure have been explained by my physician.

7. Any tissues or parts surgically removed may be disposed of by the hospital or physician in accordance with accustomed practice.

I certify this form has been fully explained to me, that I have read it or have had it read to me, that the blank spaces have been filled in, and that I understand its contents.

DATE: _____ TIME: _____ A.M. / P.M.

_____
PATIENT/OTHER LEGALLY RESPONSIBLE PERSON SIGN

WITNESS: _____

_____
RELATIONSHIP OF LEGALLY RESPONSIBLE PERSON TO PATIENT

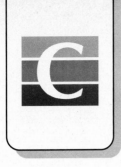

Accepted Abbreviations and Descriptive Terms for Charting

ABBREVIATIONS TYPICALLY USED IN CHARTING

Abbreviation	Word or phrase	Abbreviation	Word or phrase
abd.	abdomen	I & O	intake and output
a.c.	before meals	IM	intramuscular
ad lib	freely, as desired	IV	intravenous
amt.	amount	Kg.	kilogram
AP	apical pulse	KUB	kidneys, ureters, and bladder
aq.	water	L	left
b.(2) i.d.	2 times a day	l.	liter
BP	blood pressure	lab.	laboratory
B.R.P.	bathroom privileges	LBP	low back pain
C or Cent.	centigrade	LLQ	left lower quadrant—abdomen
c̄	with		
caps.	capsule	LP	lumbar puncture
cc.	cubic centimeter	LUQ	left upper quadrant—abdomen
CHF	congestive heart failure		
cm.	centimeter	MI	myocardial infarction
D.C.	discontinue	mcg	microgram
ECG	electrocardiogram	mg.	milligram
ED	emergency department	ml	milliliter
EEG	electroencephalogram	MVA	motor vehicle accident
ENT	ear, nose, and throat	noct.	at night
ER	emergency room	N.P.O.	nothing by mouth
fld.	fluid	N.S.	normal saline solution
G.B.	gallbladder	Obs.	obstetrics
GI	gastrointestinal	OD	right eye
Gm.	gram	O.J.	orange juice
gtt.	drop, drops	O.P.C.	outpatient clinic
GU	genitourinary	OR	operating room
Gyn.	gynecology	OS	left eye
(H)	hypodermically	P	after
H. or hrs.	hour, hours	p.c.	after meals
H₂O	water	pH	hydrogen ion concentration
HA	headache	P.O.	by mouth
Hb	hemoglobin	P.P.	postprandial, after meals
H.S.	bedtime	p.r.n.	when necessary, as needed
		q.h.	every hour

Abbreviation	Word or phrase	Abbreviation	Word or phrase
q.2.h.	every 2 hours	ss.	one half
q.(4) i.d.	4 times a day	stat.	at once
q.s.	sufficient quantity	t.(3) i.d.	3 times a day
RBC	red blood count	TPR	temperature, pulse, respiration
RUQ	right upper quadrant—abdomen	URI	upper respiratory in-fection
Rx	therapy		
s̄	without	UTI	urinary tract infection
SOB	short of breath	WBC	white blood count
spec.	specimen	W.C.	wheelchair
SQ	subcutaneous	wt.	weight
		×	times

DESCRIPTIVE TERMS TYPICALLY USED IN CHARTING

Area of concern	Factor to be charted	Suggested terms to use
Abdomen	Hard, boardlike	Hard, rigid
	Appears swollen, rounded	Distended
	Soft, flabby, flat	Relaxed, flaccid, flat
		1. Right hypochondriac region
		2. Epigastric region
		3. Left hypochondriac region
		4. Right lumbar region
		5. Umbilical region
		6. Left lumbar region
		7. Right iliac region
		8. Hypogastric region
		9. Left iliac region

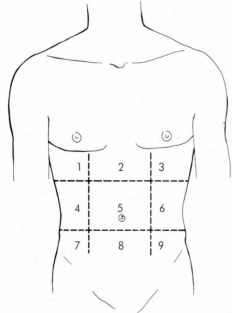

Area of concern	Factor to be charted	Suggested terms to use
Areas or regions of the abdomen		1. Right upper quadrant 2. Left upper quadrant 3. Right lower quadrant 4. Left lower quadrant

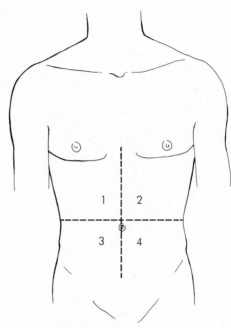

Area of concern	Factor to be charted	Suggested terms to use
Amounts	Large amount	Excessive, profuse, copious
	Moderate amount	Moderate, usual
	Small amount	Scanty, slight
General appearance	Thin and undernourished	Emaciated
	Fat, greatly overweight	Obese
	Seems very sick	Acutely ill
Appetite	Loss of appetite	Anorexia
	Refuses to eat	Refused food (state reason)
Mental attitude	Has "don't care" attitude	Apathetic
	Afraid, worried	Anxious, apprehensive
	Feeling blue, sad	Depressed
		Other characteristic terms: anxiety, defiance, anger, pain, boredom, worry, happiness, dissatisfaction, irritability
Areas of the back	Small of the back	Lumbar region
	End of spine	Sacral region
	Buttocks	Gluteal area

Area of concern	Factor to be charted	Suggested terms to use
Bleeding	Very little	Oozing
	Nosebleed	Epistaxis
	Blood in vomitus	Hematemesis
	Blood in urine	Hematuria
	Coughing or spitting up blood	Hemoptysis
	Bleeding stopped	Hemorrhage controlled
Breathing	Breathing	Respiration
	Act of inhaling	Inspiration
	Act of exhaling	Expiration
	Difficulty in breathing	Dyspnea, dyspneic
	Unable to breathe lying down	Orthopnea
	Cessation of breathing for short periods	Apnea
	Rapid breathing	Hyperpnea
	Increasing dyspnea with periods of apnea	Cheyne-Stokes respiration
	Large amount of air inspired or expired	Deep breathing
	Small amount of air inspired or expired	Shallow breathing
	Abnormal variations in rhythm	Irregular respiration
Chill	Blanket applied to keep warm	External heat applied
	Severity (degree of)	Severe, moderate, slight
	Duration	Persistent or short duration
	Came on suddenly	Sudden onset
Level of consciousness	Fully conscious, aware of surroundings	Alert, fully conscious
	Only partly conscious	Stuporous
	Unconscious, but can be aroused	Semicomatose
	Unconscious, cannot be aroused	Comatose

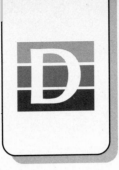

Radiology Department
Safety Procedures

ELECTRICAL SAFETY

1. All electrical equipment and appliances used within the hospital must be approved by Underwriters Laboratories and must have grounded (three-pronged) plugs.
2. All electrical outlets will be inspected periodically for adequate grounding and proper connection.
3. Any electrical problems (e.g., frayed wires, poor connections, loose plugs) are to be reported to the chief technologist immediately.
4. The chief technologist will take immediate steps to correct any problems that relate to electrical safety. Work orders relating to safety hazards shall be clearly marked "SAFETY HAZARD."
5. Carbon dioxide fire extinguishers will be available within the radiology department and are the only type to be used for electrical fires.

RADIATION SAFETY

1. Radiology personnel *will not* hold patients for radiographic examination. If it is necessary that a child or other patient be physically restrained for a radiographic procedure, a family member will be asked to help. In the absence of a family member, a person from nursing service who is responsible for the patient's care and who is not routinely exposed to ionizing radiation will be asked to hold the patient. Persons holding patients for exposures will be supplied with a lead apron and lead gloves and will be instructed to stand in such a position as to receive as little primary radiation as possible. Pregnant women will not be permitted to hold patients during exposures.
2. All personnel will stand behind the lead barrier (in the control booth) during x-ray exposures. Technologists will not lean out of the control booth or reach outside the booth while making exposures.
3. Whenever possible, the cords on exposure controls will be short so that it is impossible to make an exposure from outside the control booth.
4. Warning will be given and opportunity to leave the room before an ex-

posure is made. No exposure will be made while another person is in the room unnecessarily. If any person (employee or physician) repeatedly refuses to leave the room while an exposure is being made, the situation will be reported to the chief radiologist.

5. All personnel will wear lead aprons during fluoroscopic procedures and while making exposures in surgery or with the mobile x-ray units.

6. Unless a "wrap around" apron is worn, personnel must face the radiation field at all times during fluoroscopy and mobile x-ray exposures.

7. All personnel working in and around radiation areas will wear radiation monitor badges. Badges will be worn at collar level and will not be covered by lead aprons.

8. Badge service will be provided by the hospital for all appropriate personnel. Films from badges will be collected monthly and sent to a qualified radiation laboratory for evaluation. Results will be posted monthly for review by personnel and will be kept on file permanently.

9. All women of child-bearing age will be queried whether they might be pregnant before proceeding with any examination. Whenever possible, examinations of the abdomen and/or pelvis of women of child-bearing age will be done within the first 10 days after the onset of menstruation. If pregnancy is possible, the chief radiologist is to be notified before proceeding with the examination. In the absence of the chief radiologist, the associate is to be notified.

10. When any radiographic examination not involving the abdomen or pelvis is done on a pregnant patient, the entire abdomen and pelvis are to be shielded with lead.

11. When any examination is performed on the trunk or lower extremity of any patient under the age of 55, the gonad area is to be shielded with lead, provided that careful shielding will not obscure the subject of the examination.

CARE OF EQUIPMENT

1. All radiography equipment must be maintained in good working order. Preventive maintenance schedules will be posted and followed for all major equipment.

2. Any mechanical or electrical problem will be reported immediately to the chief technologist or supervisor. Necessary precautions will be taken to prevent further damage.

3. All personnel will care for equipment by routine cleaning, avoiding physical abuse, and following guidelines of preventive maintenance.

GENERAL PATIENT SAFETY

NOTE: Any unusual occurrence, accident, or incident affecting the safety of a patient, visitor, or staff member is to be reported immediately to the chief technologist or chief radiologist.

1. Whenever a patient is lying on a stretcher, the side rails must be raised into the "up" position.

2. Footrests on wheelchairs must be moved aside whenever a patient is helped into or out of a wheelchair.

3. Patients who are under 12 years of age, sedated, incoherent, unconscious, or otherwise of questionable responsibility will not be left unattended.

4. Patients who have not stood or walked since an accident, surgery, or illness will not be allowed to stand or walk in the radiology department. Such patients will be transported by stretcher and lifted onto the radiographic table. They will be provided with a bedpan instead of being allowed to walk to the bathroom, even if they believe they are capable of walking.

5. Pneumatic splints and other radiolucent splinting devices are not to be removed by radiology department personnel except on the radiologist's direct order after review of initial survey films.

6. Critically ill patient safety
   a. Any critically ill patient will have a nurse and/or physician in attendance while the patient is in the radiology department.
   b. An adequate supply of personnel will be in attendance as needed.
   c. Necessary lifesaving devices (oxygen, emergency kit, medications, suction, etc.) will be available.

7. Radiology procedures outside the department
   a. Make certain equipment is in good operating condition, both electrically and mechanically.
   b. Use technical factors to produce quality films within equipment limits and patient safety requirements.
   c. Protect the patient, personnel, and self with proper shielding and collimation.
   d. Observe all principles of sterile technique when in isolation or surgery.

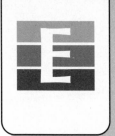

Incident Report Form

Redland Valley Hospital	(Patient ID Plate)
INCIDENT REPORT	

Incident Date:_____Time:_____

Victim: ☐ Patient   ☐ Employee   ☐ Visitor   ☐ Other
Name:_____ Address_____ Phone_____

Location:_____
Description of incident:_____
_____
_____
_____

Action taken:_____
_____
_____
_____

Seen by Physician: ☐ Yes   ☐ No   Physician Name:_____

Action taken:_____
_____
_____
_____

Name:_____ Witness:_____
Signature:_____ Signature:_____
Title:_____ Witness:_____
                          Signature:_____

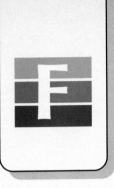

Radiology Department
Infection Control
Procedures

I. Routine departmental cleaning
   A. Floors
      1. Wet mop *daily* using germicidal solution.
      2. Strip and scrub weekly using germicidal solution, followed by waxing and buffing.
   B. Counters and surfaces frequently contacted by personnel who handle patients:
      1. wipe down twice daily using dilute bleach*.
         (NOTE: These surfaces are to include counters and work areas in radiography rooms, counters surrounding reception desk, darkroom counters, and counters in film-viewing areas.)
   C. Closed storage areas containing linen and nonsterile medical supplies: wipe shelves and doors weekly with dilute bleach*.
   D. Storage areas containing sterile supplies.
      1. Dust daily using cloth with dilute bleach*.
      2. Wash weekly, removing all items from shelves, using Vesphene germicide.
         (NOTE: Check expiration dates on all sterile supplies at time of weekly cleaning and resterilize items as needed.)
   E. Lead aprons and gloves
      1. Wash weekly using dilute bleach*.
      2. Wash with dilute bleach* following contact with blood or body fluids.
   F. Portable x-ray machines
      1. Wash weekly using dilute bleach*. Pay particular attention to the x-ray tube, tube arm, and collimator, which are suspended over the patient, as well as those parts that contact the floor, such as cables and wheels.
      2. Wipe thoroughly with dilute bleach* before entering surgery, newborn nursery, or patient room designated for protective isolation.
   G. X-ray machines and tables

---

*Sodium hypochlorite mixed 1 part to 10 parts water.

1. Thoroughly wet radiography table top with dilute bleach* and wipe down after each patient.
2. Change pillowcases, using clean linen for each patient.
3. Dust daily the overhead tube, spot film devices, image intensifiers, and television monitors.
4. Dust weekly the overhead tracks for ceiling-mounted equipment using a vacuum cleaner.
5. Wash weekly the control stands, spot film devices, and the entire radiography table with Vesphene germicide.

H. Wheelchairs and stretchers
1. Thoroughly wash each wheelchair and stretcher with dilute bleach* weekly.
2. Wipe down stretcher mattresses and patient contact areas of wheelchairs with alcohol daily.
3. Wash down wheelchairs or stretchers used for isolation patients with Vesphene immediately following use.
4. Wipe down wheelchairs or stretchers contaminated with patient secretions or excretions with dilute bleach* before being reused.

II. Personnel practices
A. Handwashing—personnel are instructed to wash hands at following times.
1. On reporting for duty
2. Between examinations of patients
3. Before touching the area surrounding the patient's mouth and nose
4. After contact with the patient's excretions or secretions
5. Before eating
6. After personal use of the toilet
7. After blowing or wiping the nose
8. On entering and leaving isolation areas or handling articles for isolation areas
9. After handling dressings, sputum containers, urinals, catheters, or bedpans
10. On completing duty

B. All personnel are to observe body substance precautions (see Appendix G) whenever contact with blood or body fluids is possible.

C. Good personal hygiene—personnel are directed to practice the following.
1. Bathe and wash hair regularly.
2. Wear clean uniforms and duty shoes.
3. Pay particular attention to frequently overlooked items of personal cleanliness, such as fingernails, watchbands, intricate jewelry, and shoelaces.
4. Change clothing that is soiled in the process of patient care before continuing work.
5. Not report for duty when affected by the following.
   a. Contagious skin diseases
   b. Acute upper respiratory infections
   c. Any other communicable diseases

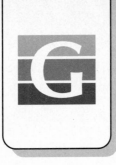

Isolation Guidelines*

CATEGORY-SPECIFIC ISOLATION PRECAUTIONS

Strict isolation

Precautions
1. Masks are indicated for all persons entering room.
2. Gowns are indicated for all persons entering room.
3. Gloves are indicated for all persons entering room.
4. *Hands must be washed after touching the patient or potentially contaminated articles and before taking care of another patient.*
5. Articles contaminated with infective material should be discarded or bagged and labeled before being sent for decontamination and reprocessing.

Diseases requiring strict isolation
Diphtheria, pharyngeal
Lassa fever and other viral hemorrhagic fevers, such as Marburg virus disease (Private room with special ventilation indicated.)
Plague, pneumonic
Varicella (chickenpox)
Zoster, localized in immunocompromised patient, or disseminated

Contact isolation

Precautions
1. Masks are indicated for those who come close to patient.
2. Gowns are indicated if soiling is likely.
3. Gloves are indicated for touching infective material.
4. *Hands must be washed after touching the patient or potentially contaminated articles and before taking care of another patient.*
5. Articles contaminated with infective material should be discarded or bagged and labeled before being sent for decontamination and reprocessing.

*From Centers for Disease Control: CDC guidelines for isolation precautions in hospitals, *Infect Control* 4(4):250, 1983.

Diseases or conditions requiring contact isolation
Acute respiratory infections in infants and young children
Conjunctivitis, gonococcal, in newborns
Diphtheria, cutaneous
Endometritis, group A *Streptococcus*
Furunculosis, staphylococcal, in newborns
Herpes simplex, disseminated, severe primary or neonatal
Impetigo
Influenza, in infants and young children
Multiply resistant bacteria, infection, or colonization (any site) with any of the
   following:
   1. Gram-negative bacilli resistant to all aminoglycosides that are tested
   2. *Staphylococcus aureus* resistant to methicillin
   3. *Pneumococcus* resistant to penicillin
   4. *Haemophilus influenzae* resistant to ampicillin and chloramphenicol
   5. Other resistant bacteria may be included in this isolation category if they
      are judged by the infection control team to be of special clinical or epide-
      miological significance.
Pediculosis
Pharyngitis, infectious, in infants and young children
Pneumonia, viral, in infants and young children
Rabies
Rubella, congenital and other
Scabies
Scalded skin syndrome (Ritter's disease)
Skin, wound, or burn infection, major (draining and not covered, or dressing
   does not adequately contain the purulent material), including those infected
   with *Staphylococcus aureus* or group A *Streptococcus*
Vaccinia (generalized and progressive eczema vaccinatum)

Respiratory isolation

Precautions
   1. Masks are indicated for those who come close to patient.
   2. Gowns are not indicated.
   3. Gloves are not indicated.
   4. *Hands must be washed after touching the patient or potentially contaminated arti-*
      cles and before taking care of another patient.
   5. Articles contaminated with infective material should be discarded or
      bagged and labeled before being sent for decontamination and reprocess-
      ing.

Diseases requiring respiratory isolation
   Epiglottitis, *Haemophilus influenzae*
   Erythema infectiosum
   Measles
   Meningitis
      Bacterial, etiology unknown

Haemophilus influenzae, known or suspected
Meningococcal, known or suspected
Meningococcal pneumonia
Mumps
Pertussis (whooping cough)
Pneumonia, *Haemophilus influenzae,* in children (any age)

AFB (acid-fast bacilli) isolation
Precautions
1. Masks are indicated only when patient is coughing and does not reliably cover mouth.
2. Gowns are indicated only if needed to prevent gross contamination of clothing.
3. Gloves are not indicated.
4. *Hands must be washed after touching the patient or potentially contaminated articles and before taking care of another patient.*
5. Articles should be discarded, cleaned, or sent for decontamination and reprocessing.

Diseases requiring AFB isolation.   This isolation category is for patients with current pulmonary tuberculosis (TB) who have a positive sputum smear or a chest x-ray appearance that strongly suggests current (active) TB. Laryngeal TB is also included in this category. In general, infants and young children with pulmonary TB do not require isolation precautions because they rarely cough and their bronchial secretions contain few AFB compared with adults with pulmonary TB. To protect the patient's privacy, the instruction card is labeled *AFB* (acid-fast bacilli) rather than *Tuberculosis Isolation.*

Enteric precautions
Precautions
1. Masks are not indicated.
2. Gowns are indicated if soiling is likely.
3. Gloves are indicated for touching infective material.
4. *Hands must be washed after touching the patient or potentially contaminated articles and before taking care of another patient.*
5. Articles contaminated with infective material should be discarded or bagged and labeled before being sent for decontamination and reprocessing.

Diseases requiring enteric precautions
Amebic dysentery
Cholera
Coxsackievirus disease
Diarrhea, acute illness with suspected infectious etiology
Echovirus disease
Encephalitis (unless known not to be caused by enteroviruses)
Enterocolitis caused by *Clostridium difficile* or *Staphylococcus aureus*

Enteroviral infection
Gastroenteritis caused by:
  Campylobacter species
  Cryptosporidium species
  Dientamoeba fragilis
  Escherichia coli (enterotoxic, enteropathogenic, or enteroinvasive)
  Giardia lamblia
  Salmonella species
  Shigella species
  Vibrio parahaemolyticus
  Viruses, including Norwalk and rotavirus
  Yersinia enterocolitica
  Unknown etiology but presumed to be an infectious agent
Hand, foot, and mouth disease
Hepatitis, viral, type A
Herpangina
Meningitis, viral (unless known not to be caused by enteroviruses)
Necrotizing enterocolitis
Pleurodynia
Poliomyelitis
Typhoid fever *(Salmonella typhi)*
Viral pericarditis, myocarditis, or meningitis (unless known not to be caused by enteroviruses)

Drainage/secretion precautions

Precautions

1. Masks are not indicated.
2. Gowns are indicated if soiling is likely.
3. Gloves are indicated for touching infective material.
4. *Hands must be washed after touching the patient or potentially contaminated articles and before taking care of another patient.*
5. Articles contaminated with infective material should be discarded or bagged and labeled before being sent for decontamination and reprocessing.

Diseases requiring drainage/secretion precautions.   Infectious diseases included in this category are those that result in production of infective purulent material, drainage, or secretions, unless the disease is included in another isolation category that requires more rigorous precautions. (If you have questions about a specific disease, see the listing of infectious diseases in *Guideline for Isolation Precautions in Hospitals,* Table A, *Disease-Specific Isolation Precautions.**)

The following infections are examples of those included in this category provided they are *not* (1) caused by multiply resistant microorganisms; (2) major (draining and not covered by a dressing or dressing does not adequately contain the drainage) skin, wound, or burn infections, including those caused by

---

*Not included here.

Staphylococcus aureus or group A *Streptococcus;* or (3) gonococcal eye infections in newborns. See *Contact Isolation* if the infection is one of these three.

Abscess, minor or limited
Burn infection, minor or limited
Conjunctivitis
Decubitus ulcer, infected, minor or limited
Skin infection, minor or limited
Wound infection, minor or limited

Body substance precautions

Precautions

1. Masks are not indicated.
2. Gowns are indicated if soiling with blood or body fluids is likely.
3. Gloves are indicated if touching blood or body substances.
4. *Hands should be washed immediately if they are potentially contaminated with blood or body fluids and before taking care of another patient.*
5. Articles contaminated with blood or body fluids should be discarded or bagged and labeled before being sent for decontamination and reprocessing.
6. Care should be taken to avoid needle-stick injuries. Used needles should not be recapped or bent; they should be placed in a prominently labeled, puncture-resistant container designated especially for such disposal.
7. Blood spills should be cleaned up promptly with a solution of 5.25% sodium hypochlorite diluted 1:10 with water.

Diseases requiring body substance precautions

Acquired immunodeficiency syndrome (AIDS)
Arthropod-borne viral fevers (for example, dengue, yellow fever, and Colorado tick fever)
Babesiosis
Creutzfeldt-Jakob disease
Hepatitis B (including HBsAg antigen carrier)
Hepatitis, non-A, non-B
Leptospirosis
Malaria
Rat-bite fever
Relapsing fever
Syphilis, primary and secondary with skin and mucous membrane lesions

DISEASE-SPECIFIC ISOLATION PRECAUTIONS
Sample instruction card

(Front of Card)

Visitors—Report to Nurses' Station Before Entering Room

1. Private room indicated?
    _____ No
    _____ Yes

2. Masks indicated?
    _____ No
    _____ Yes for those close to patient
    _____ Yes for all persons entering room

3. Gowns indicated?
    _____ No
    _____ Yes if soiling is likely
    _____ Yes for all persons entering room

4. Gloves indicated?
    _____ No
    _____ Yes for touching infective material
    _____ Yes for all persons entering room

5. Special precautions indicated
    for handling blood?
    _____ No
    _____ Yes

6. HANDS MUST BE WASHED AFTER TOUCHING THE PATIENT OR POTENTIALLY CONTAMINATED ARTICLES AND BEFORE TAKING CARE OF ANOTHER PATIENT.

7. Articles contaminated with _____
    (infective material[s])
    should be discarded or bagged and labeled before being sent for decontamination and reprocessing.

(Back of Card)

Instructions

1. On Table B, *Disease-Specific Precautions,** locate the disease for which isolation precautions are indicated.
2. Write disease in blank space here:_____
3. Determine if a private room is indicated. In general, patients infected with the same organism may share a room. For some disease conditions, a private room is indicated if patient hygiene is poor. A patient with poor hygiene does not wash hands after touching infective material (feces, purulent drainage, or secretions), contaminates the environment with infective material, or shares contaminated articles with other patients.
4. Place a check mark beside the indicated precautions on front of card.
5. Cross through precautions that are *not* indicated.
6. Write infective material in blank space in item 7 on front of card.

*Not included here.

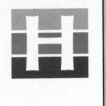

Allergy History Form

Redland Valley Hospital

(Patient ID Plate)

Iodine Contrast Agent Injection Questionaire

Name:_____ Age_____ Weight_____

Yes   No

☐   ☐   Have you ever had a reaction to iodine, iodine contrast or "x-ray dye" ?
             If Yes, describe:_____

☐   ☐   Are you allergic to any medications ?
             If Yes, list:_____

☐   ☐   Do you have any other allergies ?
             If Yes, list:____ _____

☐   ☐   Do you have asthma ?

☐   ☐   Do you have serious heart disease ?

☐   ☐   Do you have multiple myeloma, sickle cell disease, polycythemia
             or pheochromocytoma ?

☐   ☐   Do you have severe kidney disease ?

☐   ☐   Do you have diabetes with kidney complications ?

Patient signature:_____ Date:_____

Index

Coramine; *see* Nikethamide
Corynebacterium diphtheriae, 102
Coumadin; *see* Warfarin
Co-workers, communication with, 44-51
"Crash carts," 168-169
Credentialing, 7-9
Credentials
  institutional, 7-8
  for radiographers, 8-9
Cricothyroid method for instillation of contrast
      medium in bronchography, percutaneous,
      236
Crisis intervention, 26
CT; *see* Computed tomography
Cyanosis as guide to patient status, 85-86
Cysto-Conray; *see* Iothalamate meglumine
Cystografin; *see* Diatrizoate meglumine
Cystography, 221-223
Cystourethrograms, voiding, 221
  iodinated contrast media for, 217

D

Deaf patient, communication with, 38-39
Death
  dealing with, 27-29
  with dignity, patient's right to, 18
Decubitus ulcers, 71
Defibrillator, 172, 173
Dehiscence, wound, 185
Demerol; *see* Meperidine
Denial in grieving process, 27
Depressants, cardiac, effects and examples of,
      136
Depression in grieving process, 28
Dermatologist, functions of, 2
Descriptive terms used in charting, 277-279
Dexamethasone, 170
Dexedrine; *see* Amphetamines
Dextromethorphan hydrobromide, 136
Diabetes, 187
Diabetic coma, 186-188
Diabinese; *see* Chlorpropamide
Diagnosis and radiographer, 13-14
Diagnostic medical sonography, 249
Diagnostic studies
  multiple, scheduling and sequencing of,
      191-192
  sequencing order for, guide to, 192
Diagnostic ultrasound, 249
Diamox; *see* Acetazolamide
Diaphoresis, 86
Diastolic blood pressure, 94
Diatrizoate meglumine, 213, 214, 215
  for cystography, 222
  and diatrizoate sodium, 213, 214
    for CT studies of abdomen, 244

Diatrizoate meglumine—cont'd
  and diatrizoate sodium—cont'd
    for gastrointestinal examinations, 200
    for intravenous urography, 220
  for intravenous urography, 220
  and iodipamide meglumine, 215
  for retrograde pyelography, 227
Diatrizoate meglumine injection; *see* Diatrizoate
      meglumine
Diatrizoate sodium, 213, 215
  for gastrointestinal examinations, 200
Diazepam, 137, 139-140, 170
Diet before barium studies of gastrointestinal
      tract, 193
Digital subtraction angiography, 240
  iodinated contrast media for, 216
Digital thermometer to check patient's
      temperature, 87-88
Digitalis, 136, 170
Dignity, death with, patient's right to, 18
Digoxin, 170
Dilantin; *see* Phenytoin
Dilution, microbial, 101
Dionosil; *see* Propyliodone
Diphenhydramine hydrochloride, 136, 138, 170
  for reaction to contrast media, 183
Direct contact, disease transmission by, 104
Director, hospital, 3-4
Disaster plan, 188-189
Disasters, 188-189
Discography, iodinated contrast media for, 217
Disease; *see also* specific disease
  lung, position for patient with, 94
  transmission of, 104-105
    preventing, 105-107
Disease-specific isolation precautions, 291
Disposable thermometer to check patient's
      temperature, 89
Disposal of contaminated waste, 111-114
Diuretics, effects and examples of, 136
Diuril; *see* Chlorothiazide
"Do not resuscitate" order, 18
Doppler ultrasound, 249
Doppler unit to monitor blood pressure, 94
Dopram; *see* Doxapram
Dosage, medication, measurement of, 141-142
Double-contrast barium enema, 205-206
Double-contrast upper gastrointestinal study,
      206, 208
Down's syndrome, communication with patient
      with, 39
Doxapram, 137
Drainage, closed chest, radiography of patient
      with, 262
Drainage/secretion precautions, 289-290
"Draw" sheet for patient transfer, 70